# INSTITUTION AND OUTCOME

*A Comparative Study of Psychiatric Hospitals*

# INSTITUTION AND OUTCOME

*A Comparative Study of Psychiatric Hospitals*

*by*

LEONARD P. ULLMANN

*University of Illinois*

PERGAMON PRESS

OXFORD · LONDON · EDINBURGH · NEW YORK
TORONTO · SYDNEY · PARIS · BRAUNSCHWEIG

Pergamon Press Ltd., Headington Hill Hall, Oxford
4 & 5 Fitzroy Square, London W.1
Pergamon Press (Scotland) Ltd., 2 & 3 Teviot Place, Edinburgh 1
Pergamon Press Inc., 44–01 21st Street, Long Island City, New York 11101
Pergamon of Canada, Ltd., 6 Adelaide Street East, Toronto, Ontario
Pergamon Press (Aust.) Pty. Ltd., 20–22 Margaret Street, Sydney, N.S.W.
Pergamon Press S.A.R.L., 24 rue des Écoles, Paris 5e
Vieweg & Sohn GmbH, Burgplatz 1, Braunschweig



First edition 1967

Library of Congress Catalog Card No. 67-15605

*Printed in Great Britain by A. Wheaton & Co., Ltd., Exeter*

3126/67

*In memory of my father,*

SIEGFRIED ULLMANN

# *Contents*

# *Introduction*

FOLLOWING the historic work of Philippe Pinel in France and the Tuke family in England, the early years of the nineteenth century saw the development in this country of a number of small mental hospitals. By all contemporaneous accounts, these hospitals achieved remarkable success in the treatment and restoration to society of mentally ill persons. The placement of mentally disordered persons in mental hospitals became established public policy.

By the end of the century our mental hospitals had become enormous, impersonal, end-of-the-road institutions, understaffed and overcrowded. They served the purpose of locking the mentally ill away from the community. The original therapeutic objectives and the attendant success achieved in restoring patients to the community had vanished along the way. The story, too long to be detailed here, is a noteworthy and distressing example of social retrogression.

Progress in the public care of the hospitalized mentally ill became visible again after the First World War. It began to be noteworthy after the Second World War, in part as a result of the medical program of the Veterans Administration. In general the VA hospitals were much better staffed than the state hospitals and proved superior to them. In the 1950's the Veterans Administration built several psychiatric hospitals of relatively small size, in a pattern of architecture with which the name of Dr. Paul Haun is associated. These hospitals contained small nursing units, required more staff than the old style hospitals and cost approximately twice as much per patient for daily care. Questions about what return the taxpayer got on the extra cost of care in these hospitals led to the Veterans Administration Psychiatric Evaluation Project (PEP).

This project chose the successful restoration of the veteran patient to the community as the most acceptable criterion of hospital success. In comparing 12 hospitals, quite extensive measures were used to control the possibility that the different degrees of success of different hospitals might be due to differences in the kinds of patients admitted to these hospitals. These controls discredited the claim that observed differences in hospital success were to be accounted for in observable differences in the types of patients received by different hospitals. Dr. Ullmann, with Dr. Lee Gurel, secured from the VA routinely collected data on all VA psychiatric hospitals. Dr. Ullmann, comparing the result of his study of routinely collected statistical data with the data specially collected in the 12 hospitals in the PEP study, was able to develop and effectively to validate a method of hospital comparison based on routinely collected data, and to extend it to 30 psychiatric hospitals. The result is, I believe, both startling and highly valuable.

In explaining his findings, Dr. Ullmann undertakes some consideration of social organization and specifically of the characteristics of bureaucratic organization. We must recognize that uncoordinated individual efforts could not meet the social problem of mental illness. Organization is necessary. Let it be noted that it was the bureaucratic nature of the Veterans Administration Department of Medicine and Surgery which made it possible for Dr. Ullmann to secure the data on which this revealing report is based. However, it is common knowledge that bureaucratic control has weaknesses as well as strengths. The report concludes that the bureaucratic organizational pattern has very serious deficiencies in meeting some kinds of human needs, including the needs of the psychiatric hospital.

Correlations measure association. They do not establish the fact nor the direction of causation. However, Dr. Ullmann presents massive and discriminating evidence to support his inferences. Those who would reject these inferences face a responsibility to present a reasonable alternative interpretation of the findings of this study also adequate to account for the data. This is no simple task.

RICHARD L. JENKINS, M.D.
*Department of Psychiatry*
*University of Iowa*

# *Preface*

> "I regard waste as the continuing enemy of our society and the prevention of waste—waste of resources, waste of lives, or waste of opportunity—to be the most dynamic of the responsibilities of government."
>
> (LYNDON B. JOHNSON)

AT THIS time half of all hospital beds in the United States are devoted to psychiatric patients. This state of affairs represents an enormous societal investment in physical structures and skilled personnel. It represents a loss of productivity, liberty, personal dignity, and, all too often, hope for a significant portion of our population. To the extent that behaviour is a function of the immediate environment, the effectiveness of psychiatric hospitals can be improved at little or no additional expense. The first object of this book is to present as tight an evaluation as my limited data and skills permit of the correlation between various hospital characteristics and the effectiveness with which hospitals return psychiatric patients to the extra-hospital community. A second purpose is to extend psychological methods, both statistical and social reinforcement analysis, from the context of individual actions to relationships in an organizational context. It will be argued that much of the behaviour of both hospital staff and patients is affected by environmental variables such as the size of the institution. A third purpose of this undertaking is one of service: to patients, to staff, and to taxpayers. Each of these groups has an interest in psychiatric hospitals and their improvement.

The history of this work starts with the organization. After the Second World War, the Veterans Administration emphasized increasingly the professional staffing of its hospitals. New hospitals, when constructed, were designed to be smaller and even more highly staffed. These innovations led to an increased cost per patient per day, and questions were raised whether the new procedures were justified. Some of these questions came from the Bureau of the Budget while others were generated by research workers within the VA itself, notably Drs. Quinter Holsopple and Richard L. Jenkins.

Under Dr. Jenkins' able direction field staffs were recruited and starting in Autumn, 1956, data were collected at 12 VA psychiatric hospitals. Some of the findings of that study will be discussed in chapters 4 and 5 of this book. Beginning early in 1960, I proposed the collection of data to answer with a larger sample of hospitals the questions about size and staffing originally put to the VA project. With the administrative assistance of Drs. H. Martin Engle and Lee Gurel, the request found in Appendix 1 of this book was sent to 36 VA hospitals in August, 1961. While the present undertaking grew out of the VA's study of 12 hospitals, it should be explicit that this book is not a report of the VA study. Perusal of the material of the VA's "Psychiatric Evaluation Project" presented in chapters 4 and 5 of this book and fuller reports of its findings when they become available, will indicate that the sample, method of data collection, period of study, and statistical analyses are drastically different from those of the present work. In addition, I have surveyed the psychiatric and sociological literature in order to develop a firmer rationale for the major hypotheses and to place the study of psychiatric hospitals within the context of psychological theory.

In organizing the findings, I was led to try to make sense of the psychiatric hospital environment in which I had worked for a decade. While this took me away from my data, it led me to study material on bureaucracy and social organization. As a psychologist, I obtained an experience similar to that of a rat on first reading Skinner. The system of VA psychiatric hospitals I had worked in and studied was not novel but displayed many crucial characteristics common to bureaucratic organizations.

While influenced and excited by sociological inquiries, the method employed, for better or worse, was psychological. I was an employee of the system and not a participant observer. If I had to designate my status for sociologists, it would be to ask them to treat me as an informant. The basic data uses a statistical criterion of evidence and does so for characteristics across hospitals. As noted above, first and foremost I wished to investigate thoroughly limited, specific variables. I used hospitals as subjects and procedures common to psychologists studying individual differences. A second difference between the present work and sociological studies is that I developed limited hypotheses based on available literature and after computing my data set forth additional discussions and hypotheses. The difference between my procedure and more usual forms of sociological inquiry can be seen by contrasting the present effort with the excellent recent discussion of methodology by Strauss *et al.* (1964). A final difference is that I use a social reinforcement framework as a model when formulating both patient and staff behavior. Accurate observations will lead to the description of the same phenomena, but different disciplines will provide different names. For example, my concept of "reinforcement" is very similar to Homans' concept of "value." To the extent that the present effort touches upon areas within the provinces of sociology, political science, social psychology, and psychiatry, particular terms will seem misnomers to some members of one discipline or another. I can only ask the professional reader to hearken to the behaviour under discussion. This problem may become acute because I will frequently use the reports of workers from other disciplines to extend my own observations. My limitations as a psychologist using a particular form of inquiry and my involvement as a member of the organization makes necessary this procedure which unfortunately places a more than usual burden on the reader.

While the difficulties in the present work cannot be glossed over, the problem dealt with is one of great importance. The 30 hospitals of the focal study reported in chapters 6 and 7 represented at that time a daily expenditure for patient care of over half a million dollars. Of greater import was that human beings were deprived of fundamental liberties and social rights. The 30 hospitals represented an average daily patient load of 43,577. Every professional person, whether he is engaged in therapy or research, bears the burden that to the extent he fails to do his utmost he is responsible for the continuing degradation of his fellow human beings.

Beyond the desire to know for the sake of knowing and the investigation of the influence of a major aspect of the environment, the study of organizations offers insights into the roots of much of our own behavior in mid-twentieth century America. I hope that the present work will provide a worthwhile addition to a body of knowledge characterized by remarkable similarities underlying remarkable external differences.

It is obvious that this study would not have been possible without the cooperation of the Veterans Administration. I would like to thank the many people whom I never met and whose names I do not know who compiled the raw data at the hospital level. I want to express my appreciation and admiration for the Veterans Administration executives who permitted an independent study of their organization. This is but one measure of their dedication to service for patients. Another indication is that in the time between the collection of data and the completion of this book appreciable progress has been made along some of the lines later suggested, for example, increasing use of unit systems, encouragement of therapeutic research projects, and attempts to liberalize the position classifications of professional personnel.

I would like to thank the American Medical Association for permission to reprint tables 6 through 9 and the discussion thereof which originally appeared in the Archives of General Psychiatry. The material in tables 3 and 4 of this book were previously presented in a paper read to the Western Psychological Association in 1964, and the material in table 5 was first presented in a paper read at the American Psychological Association in 1964. My tenure during the summer of 1965 on Public Health Research Grant M 6191 from the National Institute of Mental Health was crucial in the completion of the manuscript.

I am grateful to many people for their help at various stages of this work. First and foremost is my wife who gave encouragement and support throughout. Dr. Jeanne M. Giovannoni took on herself numerous tasks which would normally have fallen to me and provided time for developing and analyzing the data. Miss Vicki Gorter and Dr. Paul McReynolds provided examples of the skill and dedication on which the psychiatric hospital as a therapeutic organization is built. Finally it is a pleasure to acknowledge publicly my great personal and professional debt to Dr. Leonard Krasner.

# *Overview*

It is the current consensus of experts that psychiatric hospitals should be small and highly staffed. The final report of the Joint Commission on Mental Illness and Health (1961, pp. xxii–xxiii) has as one of its recommendations "Agree that no money will be spent to build mental hospitals of more than 1000 beds, or to add a single patient to mental hospitals presently having 1000 or more patients." The report of the Expert Committee of the World Health Organization (1953, p. 29) put the optimum size of hospitals between 250 and 400 beds.

This stress on small size has been a continuing theme in the treatment of the mentally ill. The report of the Metropolitan Commissioners in Lunacy (1844, pp. 36–38) with which the name of the seventh Earl of Shaftesbury is associated, stated in part, "From the best opinions that we have been able to collect, and from our own observations and experience, we think that it is desirable that no asylum for curable lunatics should contain more than 250 patients, and that 200 is perhaps as large a number as can be managed with the most benefit, to themselves and the public, in one establishment." (Quoted in Hunter and Macalpine, 1963, p. 927.)

Arlidge (1859, p. 104) summarized the experience and thought both of the previous 50 years and the next 100:

> In a colossal refuge for the insane, a patient may be said to lose his individuality, and to become a member of a machine so put together as to move with precise regularity and invariable routine;—a triumph of skill adapted to show how such unpromising materials as crazy men and women may be drilled into order and guided by rule, but not an apparatus calculated to restore their pristine conditions and their independent self-governing existence. In all cases admitting of recovery, or of material amelioration, a gigantic asylum is a gigantic evil, and, figuratively speaking, a manufactory of chronic insanity.

It need only to be added, that Arlidge (1859, p. 102) noted with horror the growth of hospitals into "lunatic colonies of eight or nine hundred, or even a thousand or more inhabitants."

A different recommendation of the Joint Commission on Mental Illness and Health (1961, p. xx) is "*Expenditures for public mental patient services should be doubled in the next five years—and tripled in the next ten.*" As with size, this recommendation has the support of the overwhelming majority of informed opinion, and as with building smaller hospitals, involves a decision about the use of limited funds. Unlike the variable of size, however, investment in personnel brings with it questions of what particular types of personnel.

As long as there are limited funds to accomplish many worthy social projects, it is right and proper to ask for the most stringent documentation before deciding on specific courses of action. Even within limited areas of effort, decisions must be made as to how funds, whether they remain stable or increase appreciably, might best be spent to serve the public from which they were gathered.

In obtaining data, the focus is effectiveness in treating patients. The first section will deal with this topic. A review of the literature and theoretical formulations will also be found in the first section. The second part of the book will present data dealing with 30 VA psychiatric hospitals during a full year. Institutions will be treated in the manner psychologists typically employ with people. From this work, a number of generally agreed upon concepts will be documented and a number of questions will be raised. The third section of the book will make use of the prior material to suggest ways in which hospital personnel, especially administrators, might improve the effectiveness of psychiatric hospitals.

# PART I

## *Background Material*

B

# CHAPTER 1

## *The Measure of Effectiveness*

This is a book about institutions, specifically Veterans Administration psychiatric hospitals. But it should be clear at the start that while these institutions have realities as geographical locations and as entries into fiscal and statistical tables, they are abstractions. To speak of an institution as something more than the activities and equipment of its members seems incorrect. In every case the "purposes of the institution" are the wishes of some or all of the human beings concerned. An institution such as the "hospital" is a term by which we indicate that individuals are living and working together in certain ways at a certain location. The hospital does not "treat" patients nor is the hospital "effective." Rather, when we use words such as "treatment" or "effectiveness," we refer to the result of the efforts of a group of people. It is vital that we remember that we are dealing with people who possess an ostensible common purpose that legitimizes what they do. This goal provides us with a basic evaluative measure for the analysis of situational behavior. This viewpoint is summarized in the following quotation:

> Institutions, in other words, take on reality for us *when we are looking for the fulfillment of some purpose upon a collective or multi-individual scale.* We envisage an institution when we regard human beings cooperating, in a regular and habitual fashion, toward the satisfying of some common human want. We cannot experience an institution as a reality when we merely examine or study individuals disinterestedly, but only when we try to do something *through* individuals by organizing them (or conceiving them as organized), in the direction of some ulterior common end. (Allport, 1933, p. 21.)

Given this orientation, the first matter to be discussed is the purpose of the organization. Such a purpose may be considered to legitimize behaviors by members of the organization which would otherwise be inexplicable or socially deviant. In the case of a system of hospitals supported by the federal government, the basic purpose is seemingly simple, direct, and consistent with the economic and humanitarian goals of the society. A psychiatric hospital has two *major* purposes, *protection* and *treatment*.[1]

The individual may have to be protected from himself. The person's maladjustment may be such that he cannot take care of himself, that he may do physical harm to himself, or that he may show such poor judgment as to be the victim of swindlers and lose his material possessions. In turn, society at large may need protection from the harm the individual may do others either physically or as a public nuisance. For such reasons the person may be removed from society and the hospital made to serve a custodial purpose. However, for both economic and humanitarian purposes, custodial care is inferior to treatment. Custodial care is a solution to the problem of what to do with the deviant, but one which an increasing population and a decreasing tolerance for deviance makes steadily less desirable. As the custodial population grows, the chances of remission decrease. While we shall return to this concept when we discuss the role of the psychiatric patient and the rationale for our interest in size of psychiatric hospitals, we wish to point out that custodial care is likely to lead to a vicious cycle of larger hospitalized populations, decreased remission, and hence further increases in number of hospitalized patients.

"Treatment," by removing the reasons which necessitated hospitalization, serves the purpose of protecting the patient and society. As the rate of release equals or becomes greater than the rate of intake, the negative effects of crowding are avoided. In the long run, there is the additional saving of capital investment because new hospitals need not be built. There is the possibility of a beneficent cycle in which reduced patient load leads to smaller size and an increased ratio of employees to patients and hence further improvement in the remission rate.

[1] Many purposes can be assigned to the public psychiatric hospital. Sewall and Berger (1959) for example write: "A conference was held in December of 1958 in which a number of leaders in the fields of hospital and social organization participated. This group agreed upon six goals that made the end results of psychiatric hospital operation more explicit. These six goals were custodial care, protection, social restoration, research, training and education, and a catch-all labeled administration." The present work will touch on research, training, and administrative program elements through correlations between them and measures of rapid release and high turnover. This is due in part to a view of such programs as means towards an end rather than ends in themselves and in part to grave difficulties in defining good research, training, and administration as goals in themselves.

The reader will note that in the preceding paragraph effective treatment was implicitly equated with release. This presumption must be made explicit, because we will use two related dimensions of release (rapid release and high turnover) as the operational measures of hospital effectiveness.

The equation of effective treatment and hospital release is crucial to the present research and deserves prolonged discussion. It may be argued that the person released from the hospital may return to the hospital at some later date. This is true although it should be immediately noted that if there were no releases there would be no readmissions. Two points need to be made. The first is that the measure of rapid release must include a minimum period of time in the extra-hospital community before the release is considered socially significant. We shall arbitrarily use 90 days as this minimum period of time. If a person remains in the community at least a minimum period of time, we may argue that his return to the hospital was not necessarily due to insufficient treatment, but may have been due to new social pressures. We may also argue that the period was long enough to be of value to both the patient (as a break in institutionalization) and society (as the production of treatment facilities available to another person). A second point is that the ultimate effectiveness of a psychiatric hospital lies either with the smallest ratio of time patients are in the hospital to time they reside in the community or in the smallest number of beds necessary to serve adequately a standard unit of population. That is, the hospital whose patients spend 10% of their time institutionalized after admission is more effective than the hospital whose patients are institutionalized for 50% of the time after their admission. Similarly, the hospital in which each bed serves 1000 people is more effective than the hospital in which each bed serves only a general population of 100 people. Both measures presume rapid release and high turnover. This view may be summarized by a quotation from Norton (1961):

> Some attacks seem to clear up completely; other patients do not become completely well, and in their case a fresh attack of illness or altered circumstances may bring them back to the hospital several times in the course of the illness. There seems to be no need to be disheartened by these frequent readmissions if they can be regarded as episodes in the long-term management of a patient who, if she had become ill 30 years ago, had only two chances in five of ever being discharged. At least she is now at home and often at work for the greater part of the time.

Finally, we would like to call the reader's attention to Bockoven's

(1963, pp. 56–58) discussion of the statistics of readmission after moral treatment in which nearly one-half (48 %) of the patients never had a relapse for the remainder of their lives.

It may be argued that release may not reflect the psychological state of the person leaving the hospital. At a theoretical level there is the presumption that there is some mental disease that can be cured such that the person is mentally healthy. Aside from the widespread challenge to the medical model in the field of psychiatry (Szasz, 1961, 1963) we may point to the failure of the best intentioned and ardent workers to derive an acceptable operational definition of either mental health or mental illness (Zubin, 1953; Scott, 1958). It is difficult, theoretically, to envision something on which there is no reliable definition leading to a valid prediction of post-hospital adjustment.

This difficulty is borne out at an empirical level. Adjustment to the extra-hospital community is either so complex (Freeman and Simmons, 1963) or the measures at exit from the hospital so poor or so ungermane that careful studies have had great difficulty or outright failure in making predictions of the patient's post-hospital adjustment *in terms of the patient's condition at exit.* Jones and Sidebotham (1962, pp. 126–7) summarize their data based on samples of 100 patients or more from each of three hospitals as follows: "The hospitals' estimate of condition on discharge is thus shown to bear no direct relation to patients' subsequent progress." Further, Jones and Sidebotham (1962, pp. 144–8) found that on follow-up the percentages of the "recovered" and the "relieved" working were highly similar. Parallel results were reported by Odegard (1961, p. 109, table 5) who studied Norwegian psychiatric hospitals. Of schizophrenics between 1926 and 1935 whose condition on discharge was "good," 41 % were readmitted, while the readmission rates for those whose condition on discharge was evaluated as "fair" and "poor" were 35 % and 30 % respectively. For the decade 1936 through 1945, the rates of readmission were 40 %, 38 %, and 39 % respectively for schizophrenics evaluated as in "good," "fair," and "poor" condition on discharge.

A different argument for the use of a measure of release as the criterion of effectiveness was touched on by the quotation from Arlidge in the introductory "overview." During the last 100 years, with a very few exceptions, the psychiatric hospital is more likely to have been "a manufactory of chronic insanity" than a milieu likely to improve chances of acceptable extra-hospital adjustment. While we shall return to this point in detail when discussing the effects associated with large hospital size, rapid release is socially valuable because there is the danger of the patient developing patterns of response which are rewarded within the hospital but are maladaptive outside it. Jones (1963, p. 61) summarizes the work of Barton (1959) on this point as follows:

> Dr. Barton describes "institutional neurosis" as a separate disease entity, characterized by apathy, submissiveness and inability to make decisions, and caused by custodial systems of care. He lists seven main factors in causation: loss of contact with the outside world, enforced idleness, authoritarian staff attitudes, loss of personal possessions, over-sedation, depressing surroundings, and loss of prospects for the future.

Sommer and Osmond (1961) give as symptoms of institutional care *de-individuation* which involves a reduced capacity for thought and action; *disculturation* which involves the individual acquiring institutional values and attitudes unsuited to his previous culture; *psychological or physical damage* which persists after the person has left the institution; *estrangement* which involves the extra-hospital world changing drastically during the inmate's absence; *isolation* which involves the inmate being forgotten by his friends and family; and *stimulus deprivation* which involves the person becoming accustomed to a life whose tempo differs greatly from that outside the hospital.

At this point we cannot say whether a person needs prolonged hospitalization because he is "sicker" upon admission, or whether his prolonged hospitalization in itself leads to greater difficulty in eventual release. We can, however, say that the longer a person remains in the hospital, the poorer are his chances for release (Fuller, 1930; Dunham and Weinberg, 1960; Kramer *et al.*, 1955; Malzberg, 1958; Odegard, 1961; Wanklin *et al.*, 1956). In addition we can point out that the very length of a patient's stay in the hospital may lead to the difficulties in extra-mural adjustment such as disculturation and estrangement as described by Sommer and Osmond. Long hospitalization may have an adverse effect on the attitudes of physician, patient, and relatives, all of whom have a major role in determining discharge (Freeman and Simmons, 1961). Perhaps of greatest importance is that hospitalized psychiatric patients change their behavior over time and become capable of extra-hospital adjustment. This point is made by Cooper and Early (1961) who surveyed 1012 patients of whom 85.2% had been continuously in the hospital over two years. In terms of behavior, 84.4% were not in need of custodial care and only 36.7% were totally unemployed. Cooper and Early cite other studies which obtained similar findings:

> A large proportion of all patients under care in mental hospitals show no serious disturbance of behavior, and their retention is determined largely by social factors. Cross *et al.* (1957) surveyed the chronic population of a large mental hospital, and found that most of the patients had been under care continuously for 10 years or more; only a very small proportion required constant vigilance, while about two-thirds needed only "routine care." The degree of supervision accorded seemed to depend as much on ward tradition and administrative policy as on the patients' mental disturbance.
>
> Garratt *et al.* (1958), from a study of the four Birmingham mental hospitals, found that of a large number of patients reviewed 75% needed only limited hospital facilities, while 12% needed no hospital facilities whatever, and remained in hospital for entirely social reasons. Furthermore, of the large group requiring only limited hospital facilities, 86% were fully ambulant, and 49% needed no nursing supervision in hospital.

These quotations introduce alternative criteria of benefit through treatment. As illustrated here, there may be improvement in the patient's behavior within the hospital. The value of such improvement cannot be denied. However, as in the Arlidge quotation we have previously cited, there is a distinct and frequently debatable value judgment involved in what behaviors shall be fostered as improvement within the hospital.

A second set of alternative criteria deals with quality of post-hospital adjustment and has been most thoroughly investigated by Freeman and Simmons (1963) whose work starts in many ways where the present one leaves off. Freeman and Simmons investigated patients from the point of discharge onward. Employment history and inter-personal relations can become criteria. Such criteria, however, occur only after the necessary condition of exit from the hospital. In addition, Freeman and Simmons amply demonstrate the complex variables, many beyond the scope of the hospital, which influence quality of post-hospital adjustment.

Release from psychiatric hospitals is only one of a number of socially meaningful criteria by which such hospitals may be evaluated as to effectiveness. It has been selected for the present study because it is clearly definable and reliably measured; because it is the necessary prior condition for post-hospital adjustment; and because it has a direct societal relevance in accord with the concept of treatment rather than custody.

Release from the hospital does not preclude outpatient follow-up and treatment. If anything, funds and trained personnel may become increasingly available for community psychiatric care as the salary and capital expenses of institutional treatment are reduced. Just as it may be hoped that a beneficent cycle may be initiated as the number of inpatients are reduced, so it may be hoped that savings eventually attained within the hospital will be used for work in the extra-hospital setting.

## SUMMARY

"Perhaps the minimum definition of formal organization is that collective effort is explicitly organized for specific ends" (Blau and Scott, 1962, p. 223). Rapid release and high turnover were selected as measures of the major goal of psychiatric hospitals, and this chapter was devoted to a discussion of the issues and alternatives involved in this decision.

## CHAPTER 2

# *Size*

A PRIME hypothesis of the present research is that as hospital size increases, effectiveness decreases. This hypothesis is explicit in the material previously quoted from the Joint Commission on Mental Illness and Health, the World Health Organization, and Arlidge. It is implicit in the decision by the Veterans Administration, when constructing hospitals after the Second World War, to build smaller institutions.

In this chapter we will describe neither the processes by which large size becomes associated with decreased effectiveness nor the psychiatric hospital milieu. Rather, in the sections that follow we will present some necessary general comments, a review of literature drawn from settings other than psychiatric hospitals, and a discussion of the association between size and overhead expenses.

## PRELIMINARY REMARKS

Before dealing with a review of the literature on the correlates of increasing organizational size and a formulation of the effects of larger size on both hospital staff and patients, some general remarks are necessary.

First, increasing size in and of itself is neither "good" nor "bad." In line with the orientation presented in the foregoing chapter, this could not be otherwise because "good" and "bad" imply criteria. Increases in size, productivity, and available information in our society have led to ever increasing specialization of function. This specialization itself is likely to lead to further increases in productivity and new information. Whether it be in a university laboratory or on an automobile assembly line, increased size of organization makes possible greater efficiency through specialization. Such efficiency may be measured by decreased cost per unit produced because an investment in greater selection and training is possible, or in capability itself. For example, newer, more complicated, and rarer surgical procedures are performed with a greater percentage of success at large urban than at small rural hospitals. One factor is that an increased frequency of "rare" cases increases the skill of the surgeons performing the operation.

We have touched two of the conditions under which increased size will be beneficial: (a) there is a specialized body of knowledge or procedures, and (b) the procedure is sufficiently frequent, impersonal, or redundant to present relatively few exceptions to well defined rules. We will argue later that neither of these conditions exist in the realm of the hospital treatment of psychiatric patients.

The very nature of increasing size makes more probable a number of effects which are generally considered unfavorable and which, it will be argued, are particularly detrimental in the treatment of psychiatric patients. While large size makes specialization possible and necessary it also leads to a hierarchy of authority, a system of rules, and impersonality. Specialization, hierarchy, rules, and impersonality are the four basic characteristics of bureaucratic organizations (Blau, 1956, p. 19). Larger size increases the chance of an organization showing these qualities. It is important, however, to reiterate that we will be dealing with size and its effects in terms of a special criterion, the effectiveness of treatment of hospitalized psychiatric patients.

After presenting our empirical material, we will offer suggestions as to how modifications may be made within existing structures to obviate some of the factors associated with (and *not* necessarily *caused* by) large size.

## SOME PREVIOUS STUDIES OF SIZE OF INSTITUTIONS

There is a not inconsiderable literature on the effects of increasing size. This literature ranges from work by pioneers such as Durkheim (1902), Simmel (1902), and Cooley (1909) to such recent reviews as that by Thomas and Fink (1963). The following material has as its purpose an illustration of the range of situations and criteria associated with differential size of the group and organization.

A first source of information comes from industrial settings. It should be kept in mind that much of this information relates to effects on staff; as we shall discuss, in the psychiatric hospital the dimension of size has an effect on the "objects" of production as well as on the producers. A good introductory sample of work in the field is provided by reference to Worthy's (1950) paper on organizational structure and employee morale. After 12 years' work and surveys covering over 100,000 employees, Worthy (1950, pp. 172–3) wrote:

> Our researches demonstrate that mere size is unquestionably one of the most important factors in determining the quality of employee relationships: the smaller the unit the higher the morale, and vice versa. It is clear that the closer contact between executives and rank and file prevailing in smaller organizations tends to result in friendlier, easier relationships.

Among other benefits associated with smaller size, Worthy notes that the supervisors and higher administrative officers are known personally, that there are fewer levels of supervision, less minute subdivisions of labor, and the organization operates on a face to face rather than on an impersonal, institutionalized basis.

Worthy makes a number of additional remarks which are relevant to the present discussion and foreshadow our later discussion of staff milieu in the government services. Worthy (1950, p. 176) notes that with increasing size:

> In order to achieve the necessary degree of coordination and cooperation between administratively separated functions, management is thus forced not only to build up an elaborate hierarchy of many supervisory levels, but to institute a wide variety of formal controls. Unfortunately, these controls are themselves often a source of conflict, because the individual supervisor or manager is under strong compulsion to operate in such a manner as to make a good showing in terms of the particular set of controls to which he is subject, and often he can do so only at the expense of impairing the service he is expected to render to other departments. This conflict is particularly acute when two closely related functions report up two different systems of standards and controls.

Worthy (1950) also notes that increasing size may lead to such complexity that coordination cannot occur spontaneously but must be administered. This additional requirement on upper levels of supervision is in turn reflected in anxiety and apprehension.

Worthy's work is typical in that the criteria used are variables which are presumed to affect the instrumental goals (means) by which the functional goals (ends) of the organization are achieved. It is presumed that higher morale, better coordination, and less formal supervision will lead to increased productivity. Other findings, using varying criteria of an instrumental goal nature are in agreement with Worthy. Cleland (1955) studied 82 plants and reports that small plant size allows the provision of greater personal services to the workers. This contributes to good industrial relations and therefore a small plant is more likely than a large plant to have a cohesive work force. Some indication of this is that plant size appeared to be a more significant variable in a plant's past strike history than did the union which had organized the plant or the industry in which the plant operated.

Accidents and absenteeism provide a quantifiable measure which is of value in itself and which has a strong presumptive association with productivity. For an industrial combine of 90 units, the Acton Society Trust (1953) found a clear relationship between size and morale measured in terms of sick leave, number of accidents, and length of time taken to recover from an accident. In a similar type of investigation in coalfields, lost time was found to increase with the size of the pit. A detailed study of the relationship between size and morale in five selected firms further confirmed the impression (Acton Society Trust, 1957). It was hypothesized that as firms grew in size, the management became more remote and impersonal, and, in turn, the worker developed a lack of responsibility toward his job. Revans (1957) has cited figures to show that the accident rate in American hospitals was related to the size of the hospitals. There was an increase from 2.6 accidents per million employee hours in hospitals employing less than 10 persons to 13.0 in hospitals employing over 1000 persons. Hewitt and Parfitt (1953) also found a positive relationship between size of group and voluntary absenteeism. Baumgartel and Sobol (1959) reviewed the records of 3900 nonsupervisory, non-flight airline employees and found size of work location to be positively associated with rate of absenteeism. This finding was obtained even when stratifications based on sex, seniority, age, wages, white vs. blue collar, etc., were made.

Further evidence for the association between size and absenteeism was presented by Walker (1961, p. 135) who wrote: "The correlations between numbers of all staff and the sick rates for the sick were for men, $r = 0.60$, for women, $r = 0.63$. Both correlations are too large to be attributed to chance." Walker's data were based on a study of 12 post offices all located in London (to rule out the effect of climate on respiratory ills) whose average number of staff ranged from 90 to 6410. Additional pertinent studies drawn from industrial settings are by Marriott (1949), Merrihue and Katzell (1955), and Tallachi (1960). There is some material indicative of replication of industrial findings in hospital settings. Aside from Revans' figures which were noted above, evidence for greater sociability and informal helpfulness in a general medical hospital setting is presented by Kendall (1963, p. 210, tables 7 and 8). Interns and residents at non-federal hospitals stratified by three degrees of medical school affiliation showed a greater willingness to help each other and get along together at small hospitals compared to large hospitals. Barr (1958) found correlations that were in the predicted direction but did not reach significance between the percentage of working time lost by student nurses and the number of students at the hospital and the number of beds in the hospital. A paper which is particularly germane is by Thomas (1959):

> In a study of the role conceptions and quality of performance of 109 welfare workers in small, medium, and large organizational units of a state welfare department it was found that in the smaller units there was more role consensus, greater breadth of role conception, higher ethical commitment, and better quality of work performance.

An interesting note, limited to an indirect measure of morale, but one possibly indicative of the widespread nature of the dimension of size deals with college professors. Lazarsfeld and Thielens (1958, p. 24) report that:

> In small colleges the relations among faculty members and between faculty members and administration are called unusually good by fully half the respondents. As the size of the college increases, the proportion of teachers who give their college this top rating declines, especially with regard to relations with administration.

Specifically, the decline is from 51% of respondents at the very small colleges to 21% at the very large colleges who say that there are unusually good relations between faculty and administration. This result is all the more impressive in that at larger institutions the salaries are higher, the research facilities usually better, and the teaching load lighter.

Another indirect measure of morale among professional personnel is reported by Walker (1961, p. 245) who contrasted workers at a large ministry with those at a smaller one:

> The Small Ministry's professionals were very much inclined to advise in favour of following their own careers; their estimates of their status were much higher than those of any other group, and four out of five of them placed the interest of their work first or second on their list of attractions of the job. . . .

A book by Barker *et al.* (1964) is of great importance. This is due in part to the scope and methodology of the work, and in part because the focus was on the behavior of the "products" (students, and therefore akin to patients) rather than the staff. The authors made the reasonable assumption that good facilities provide good experiences only if they are used. Participation, enthusiasm, and responsibility were viewed as necessary means to the ultimate but less well defined goal of "education." The findings of the Barker *et. al.* study reveal a negative relation between school size and individual student participation. To the degree that this is true it means that when better facilities are purchased at the expense of larger size they are discounted by lower participation by students. Instructional variety (academic scope) enlarges relatively slowly compared with growth in size: schools differing in enrolment by 100% had only a 17% median difference in instructional variety. In the smaller schools, the students were *needed* to play active roles in various behavior settings. They therefore became more involved, more active, and more responsible and participation was more widespread throughout the population.

The results of small group research by social psychologists are germane because they offer more intensive data and because much of the therapeutic and administrative work of the hospital is transacted in such groups. A prime example is work by Hare (1952, p. 267):

> As the size of a discussion group is increased from five to twelve members the degree of consensus resulting from the discussion decreases when the time for discussion is limited. . . .
>
> Because of the larger number of members in the groups of twelve, each member has less time to speak. If an individual has a chance to present his ideas, even if they are not accepted, he is generally satisfied with the results of the discussion. Consequently, since the large group members have fewer chances to speak they are less satisfied. An additional way in which a larger group limits the interaction among its members is that it increases the followers' feelings that their individual opinions are not important and therefore not worth presenting to the group.

Castore (1962) presented a theoretical analysis, which he documented with therapy groups, that as group size increases, the percentage of members with whom a relationship is possible decreases. Kelley and Thibaut (1954) note the increase of people not contributing as the size of the group increased. Bass and Norton (1951), Bales (1952), Bales and Borgatta (1955), and Taylor and Faust (1952) are authors who found increasing group size to lead to decreased efficiency of "man-minutes." Hemphill (1950) described differences between superior leaders of small (30 or fewer members) and large (over 30 members) groups. A trend to increased authoritarianism by superior leaders of large groups was noted. In a non-laboratory context LeCompte and Barker (1960) cited in Barker *et al.*, (1964, p. 34) found that in Rotary clubs and churches, as well as high schools, the size of the group tended to be negatively correlated with participation, a finding similar to that reported by Dawe (1934) for kindergarten children.

## INSTITUTIONAL SIZE, OVERHEAD, AND COORDINATION

It is often argued that increased size leads to a reduction in cost per unit produced or patient treated because functions such as organizational self-maintenance and administration can be centralized and need not be duplicated. On the other hand, it may be argued that increased size, when associated with increased specialization and bureaucratic structure, leads to such complexities that there is an increased need for coordination. For example, Wherry (1948) on the basis of a study of 145 different civilian personnel offices in the United States War Department found that in terms of fulfillment of mission, coordination of branch activities was as important, if not more important, than adequacy of the branch staff itself. The value of small size may be due in part to the reduction of task coordination, and this may in turn lead to reduced overhead.

There is empirical evidence for both lines of reasoning (Blau and Scott, 1962, pp. 226–7). Bendix (1956, p. 222), using data drawn from German industrial settings, indicates that the *percentage* of administrative salaried workers *declines* with increasing size of establishment. On the other hand, Terrien and Mills (1955) gathered data on 732 elementary school districts, 245 high school districts, and 69 unified and city school districts in California. With all three groups there were statistically significant indications that as size of organization increased, the *percentage* of employees in the administrative component *increased.* Caplow (1957, p. 484) summarizes his review as follows:

> Empirical studies suggest that the effect of size on efficiency of task performance depends upon the type of task assigned, but that increasing size is positively correlated with group stability [as defined by organizational survival over time—Ed.], the proportion of resources devoted to self-maintenance, the uniformity of organizational design, and the incidence of communication problems.

The question needs to be refined on at least two levels. The first is the type of work and its setting, as for example craft as compared to bureaucratic organizations. Anderson and Warkov (1961) offer data on this type of question. These authors found that the relative size of the administrative component decreases as size increases, but that the size of the administrative component increases as the number of places at which work is performed increases and the number of tasks performed at the same place increases.

The second level at which the question of "overhead" expense needs to be investigated is its relationship with criteria of effectiveness. It is presumed that administrative expense is wasteful. It is possible that such expenses are positively associated with effectiveness and therefore, in terms of the criteria of effectiveness, justified. Further, if this is the case, then we should break down overhead expense into its components and investigate what type of administrative activity is to be encouraged and what type is to be curtailed. Findings such as those presented in tables 10 and 14 of this volume represent a step in this direction.

## SUMMARY

In this chapter we have reviewed some of the empirical studies of size of working group and organization in non-psychiatric hospital settings. As noted by Revans (1958) and as elegantly documented by Porter and Lawler (1965, especially table 2, p. 35), increasing size usually (but not always) is associated with increased absenteeism, turnover, accidents, and labor disputes, and decreased job satisfaction and productivity. To this list we would add as of prime importance decreased participation of members (Barker *et al.*, 1964; Indik, 1963, in press).

In a later chapter discussing the hospital situation, we shall offer a description of the context in which, at least at psychiatric hospitals, large size is likely to have a negative effect. At this point, we will not offer a detailed explanation for the observed effect. Indik (1963, in press) has probably made greater contributions in this direction than any other author. He posits that structural characteristics influence the process characteristics of organizations, which in turn effect the ties that bind the individual to the organization and these bonds are directly related to behavioral outcomes. To this, as will be seen in a later chapter, we will add that environmental setting characteristics alter the behaviors that are positively reinforced. Our general view is that neither size nor bureaucratic organization are "bad" in themselves. Rather, there are particular situations in which large size and bureaucratic structure are likely to have adverse rather than beneficial effects. In the succeeding chapters, we will argue that the psychiatric hospital is such a situation because (a) it deals with humans rather than inanimate materials and (b) clear cut authority and specialization have not been achieved in the treatment of psychiatric patients.

# CHAPTER 3

## *Historical and Theoretical Considerations*

IN THE first chapter we discussed psychiatric hospitals as organizations of people, and in the second chapter the effects of one formal aspect of organizations, size, on employee behaviors. In this chapter we will discuss a number of diverse topics. First we shall give some of the historical background of the development of the public psychiatric hospitals. From our discussion of the change in psychiatric hospitals from the era of superstition to that of moral treatment to the medical model, we shall note how the view of pathology influenced the manner in which patients were treated. A second task in this chapter will therefore be an introduction of a sociopsychological model of individual behavior. After presenting our data in the second part of this book, we shall make explicit use of this model in our discussions relating our results to the behavior of *both* staff and patients.

It is crucial that we make explicit that we are dealing only with relatively large psychiatric hospitals. We will touch upon general medical hospitals only sporadically when, as in the case of Kendall (1963), there is a specific point to be made. There are many excellent histories of psychiatry (Bromberg, 1937; Deutsch, 1946; Kraepelin, 1962; Lewis, 1941; Zilboorg and Henry, 1941) and many excellent reviews, studies, and books on general hospitals such as those by Reader and Goss (1959), Georgopoulos and Mann (1962), Smith (1949), Wessen (1951), Burling, Lentz, and Wilson (1956), Freidson (1963), and Argyris (1956). It is beyond the scope of the present work to integrate this material and we will make only highly selective use of it.

Within the area of the hospital treatment of psychiatric patients, there are roughly two lines of investigation and two types of hospitals. The present work deals with public hospitals, i.e. hospitals that are supported by taxpayers and, compared to private hospitals, are relatively large. Because of this, prime material in the following discussion will come from Belknap (1956), Bockoven (1963), and Dunham and Weinberg (1960) who deal with state mental hospitals. These hospitals differ from the ones studied by Caudill (1958), Stanton and Schwartz (1954), Strauss *et al.* (1963), and Stotland and Kobler (1965) which have fewer patients, higher staffing, and a more psychoanalytic orientation. These latter studies, however, will be cited at times, because they include intensive observations of individual transactions. The focus on the individual patient necessarily supplements the more general, statistical nature of the data to be presented in this book.

Another important area deals with hospitals in the light of new progressive treatment approaches. Among the most important of these are the work of Barrabee (1951), Greenblatt *et al.* (1955), Jones (1953), and Wilmer (1958). While the ideas embodied in these books have been important in the development of current American practice in both public and private hospitals, they are peripheral to a comparative study of psychiatric hospitals. The number of cases in a study utilizing a new treatment is the number of *patients;* in the data to be presented, the number of cases, for statistical purposes, is the number of *hospitals*. The studies just mentioned for purposes of this report deal with single cases, i.e. particular hospitals. While the focal sample of this report will utilize 7212 patients to evaluate the percentage of early releases, the number of cases will be the number of hospitals at which these patients were treated, that is, 30.

## HISTORICAL BACKGROUND

In discussing the measures of effectiveness, we mentioned custodial and treatment aims. Early psychiatry was descriptive, superstitious, and reserved for the wealthy. The development of hospitals is chiefly a result of Christianity. To quote from Wessen (1951, p. 17):

> The Christian hospital was primarily structured as an institution for the practice of charity rather than as a place primarily devoted to physical healing. One of the first important Church hospitals, that of St. Basil of Caesarea (founded in 369 A.D.), set the pattern for its counterparts of the next millennium. It was "a veritable community for the sick, the aged, and orphans." The Western hospital in its very beginnings thus became a *custodial* institution.

Religious, legal, and medical concepts of the time made these places more like prisons and torture chambers than hospitals. Pinel, Tuke, Chiarugi, Reil, Langermann, and Rush deserve credit for the spread of the movement toward humanitarian treatment of the psychotic.

The efforts of these men led to the period of moral treatment in psychiatry. The first half of the nineteenth century (Dain, 1964) was marked by a remission rate which compares favorably with current efforts. The techniques of moral treatment are being returned to by contemporary psychiatrists (Harms, 1957; Rees, 1957; Walk, 1954).

Arlidge (1859, pp. 27–30) reviews various reports and writes as follows:

> Now it may be most confidently stated that insanity is a very curable disorder, if only it be brought early under treatment. American physicians go so far as to assert, that it is curable in the proportion of 90%, and appeal to their asylum statistics to establish the assertion. The Lunacy Commission of the State of Massachusetts thus wrote:—"In recent cases the recoveries amount to the proportion of 75 to 90%, of all that are submitted to the restorative process . . . ."
>
> Dr. Kirkbride, Physician to the Pennsylvania Hospital for the Insane, in his book "On the Construction and Organization of Hospitals for the Insane," says (p. 2):—"Of recent cases of insanity, properly treated, between 80 and 90% recover. Of those neglected or improperly managed, very few get well."

Arlidge notes the work at Derby Country Asylum under Hitchman and the average of 62% of admissions cured at St. Luke's Hospital, London, over a decade. Other similar reports may be cited. Jones and Sidebotham (1962, p. 124) note that "At Hanwell Asylum, it was claimed in the eighteen-thirties that 90 per cent of patients admitted were discharged 'cured.' " Dain (1964, p. 121) writes: "In the 1830's, northern superintendents claimed that out of every one hundred recently ill patients admitted to mental hospitals, eighty to ninety or more could be and sometimes were cured." Browne in 1837 (quoted in Hunter and Macalpine, 1963, p. 867) wrote: "Drs. Monro, Burrows, and Ellis, declare, however, that they cure ninety out of every hundred cases." Dunham and Weinberg (1960, p. 241) report similar figures for the Columbus, Ohio, State Hospital during the years 1839–48, while Bockoven (1963, pp. 14–15) notes parallel findings for the Hartford Retreat and Worcester State Hospital. While cultures and historical periods are not directly comparable, we might note that the poor differentiation between functional and organic disorders, the lack of effective treatment of paresis, and the paucity of admissions for neurosis and character disorders in the early nineteenth century would presumably have led to a reduction in the rate of remission. Given these results, it behooves us to investigate the variables involved in moral treatment of the insane.

In moral treatment the psychiatrist talked with the patients to find out their preoccupations; worked with their relatives; and made every effort to gain the confidence of the patients and fulfill their needs. Great attention was given to the physical setting of the hospital so that it would be cheerful, homelike, and not monotonous. Patients were treated, so far as possible, as if they were still in the enjoyment of the healthy exercise of their mental abilities. The psychiatrist also believed (Bockoven, 1963, p. 69) "in firmness and persistence in impressing on patients the idea that a change to more acceptable behavior was expected."

The hospitals were small, usually less than 200 patients in size. The superintendent and his family lived and ate with the patients who were considered part of the family and were expected, by both fellow patients and treatment personnel, to live up to the standard provided by example. The emphasis on a healthy role which was provided, expected, and reinforced, the humanitarian treatment based on a psychological model, and the expectation of improvement (Goldstein, 1962) were likely reasons for the effectiveness of moral treatment. Charles Dickens in his "American Notes" captured the spirit of moral treatment in a widely reprinted description (e.g. Greenblatt, *et al.*, 1955, pp. 409–10; Solomon, 1951, pp. 4–6).

There was a decline of moral treatment. Four factors contributed to this change which occurred from 1850 onward. The first was the building of larger, centralized state hospitals resulting from the work of Dorothea Dix. The second was the increased number of immigrants with whom the psychiatrist had difficulty communicating. The third was the success of physical medicine in overcoming many of the major diseases which had afflicted humanity from time immemorial. Perhaps the best statement of this new formulation, and the near religious belief of its major architects is presented in Jones' biography of Freud (1953, pp. 40–45). A fourth factor which, following Belknap (1956, p. 18) was probably associated with the first, was a decline in expense of treatment of the mentally ill compared with the cost of living. The citizens relieved of their responsibilities to the mentally ill by a large, isolated, and centralized institution found it easy to forget their existence and were able to settle into indifference.

Increased size and reduced expenditure led to overcrowding. Space which had been devoted to manual therapy and recreation was increasingly used to house patients. The ratio of physicians to attendants decreased. As Miller (1957, p. 11) pointed out:

As soon as the number of items of information that we must process grows too large, we resort to various ways for reorganizing and abstracting the information so that we fit it into our limited mental span. . . . The individuals are too numerous to serve as organizational foci, so we begin to put them together into subgroups in our mind and react to all members of the subgroup in a uniform, stereotyped fashion.

This trend fostered by increased size was buttressed by an emphasis on nosology.

Pinel is quoted by Bockoven (1963, p. 34): "The successful application of moral regimen exclusively gives great weight to the supposition that, in the majority of instances, there is no organic lesion of the brain nor of the cranium." Given the opposite of this, a medical model, the patient was viewed as afflicted in the same manner as patients with any organic disease. To quote Bockoven (1963, p. 84), "Once the mechanical defect concept of mental illness was adopted, no such thing as true recovery could be accepted." The patient was required to assume the role of any medically ill person (see Bloom, 1963, pp. 105 *et seq.*), a passive, submissive, quiet, untroublesome waiting for the discovery of the cure. Spontaneous remissions were looked upon with disbelief if not downright disfavor, so that the burden of proof for release was on the patient who appealed to a disbelieving judge. If no treatment were known, none could be given, and none was given. Further (Bockoven, 1963, p. 88), "The very idea of dead and decomposing brain cells carried with it the connotation of the patient's growing insensibility and unawareness of surroundings." There developed what von Mering and King (1957) call the "Legend of Chronicity." As Solomon (1951) points out, the recovery rate at Worcester State Hospital in the period 1923–32 was one-tenth what it had been for the three decades 1833–62.

A related result was the development of the aide culture. Professional staffing decreased, expectation of improvement decreased, and the goal of the hospital became one more of custody rather than treatment. The aide had as his objectives the safety and protection of his patients. His other objectives were establishing the conditions which the physician wanted and which were appropriate for medical patients: cleanliness, cooperation, quiet, and docility. The chronic, continued treatment, or back ward became characterized by inertness, listlessness, docility, and hopelessness. The physician treated the patient as the necessary locus of interesting disease and acted as if there were no effects of external events on the patients: "The attitudes of personnel, derived from such belief indicated to the patient that he lacked some essential human quality, and that his only hope for approval lay in obeying orders and deporting himself as an impersonal unquestioning individual" (Bockoven, 1963, p. 105).

To cite Belknap (1956, p. 65):

> The attendants govern both the patient's position in the patient's social system and his relations to his physician. They do this not in terms of the individual patient's psychiatric condition or needs but rather in terms of the requirements of their own social system. This fact means that the patient's first job is that of adjusting to the requirements set by the relations of the patients' system to the attendants' system. Adjustment is a critical problem for the average patient, since his contact with other personnel in the system besides the attendant and other patients amounts only to a small fraction of time through the year. Even this small amount is usually mediated through the attendant, who often interprets the patient to the ward physician, the social worker, or the occupational and recreational therapists.

The succeeding material follows closely various passages from pages 130 to 175 of Belknap's work. Given the situation in which he finds himself responsible for a large group of men, the first objective of the attendant is to give orders that will be obeyed. The aide culture developed an intricate system of rewards and penalties for patients who were helpful, troublesome, or in between these two groups. The attendant had available to him power in the form of dispensation of rewards. Privileges consisted of having the best job, sleeping in better rooms with fewer and less disturbed patients, minor luxuries such as coffee on the ward, access to privacy, going outside the ward without supervision, having access to the attendant's personal companionship and being treated in a kindly, personal, or even dignified manner, and being scheduled for such things as trips to the canteen, activities, and interviews with the physician. Punishments which could be applied by the aide included denial of the above privileges, vicious ribbing, moderate and sometimes severe corporal punishment, room seclusion and physical restraints, placement on the roster for electric shock, or transfer to a different, less desirable ward. Such elements of life as the privilege of changing one's shirt, taking a shower, or having access to better seats and a share of entertainment, were available and used by the aide.

Dunham and Weinberg (1960) report the same phenomenon and remark that the attendants respond to the patients in much the same fashion as they would respond to normal persons in a situation in which they were dominant. The implication is that this is not good because the patients are sick. We have seen from our reference to moral treatment that treating patients with the expectation of healthy behavior can be very beneficial. The difference between the aide culture and moral treatment is the short-term objective of the former. *The goal of the aide culture is the comfort of the aide and not the ultimate adjustment of the patient*, and this is indeed detrimental to the patient and the larger society whose best interests are served by effective treatment. The goal of the aide is the discharge of his duties, as he sees them, with the least effort. This goal can and does conflict with the long range goal of society which is rehabilitation and discharge. Lehrman (1961) and Goffman (1961, esp. pp. 146–69) are among authors who have remarked, as do Dunham and Weinberg, that passive, withdrawn, fearful, nonassertive behavior which rules out interpersonal rehabilitation by avoiding any involvement, is fostered by the aide culture. Dunham and Weinberg (1960, p. 48) quote a patient to the effect that, "As soon as you start holding your own and trying to stand up for yourself, the attendants say you are disturbed and want to put you down on Ward 7" (for acutely agitated patients). Again, Dunham and Weinberg (p. 122) note "They learn not to interfere with or become too personal with most other patients because in their previous social contacts, they have been rebuffed or ignored. Conversely, they learn how to thwart the baiting of other patients." Dunham and Weinberg also note (p. 120), "They had little, if anything, to do except sit continually on hard chairs and provide a minimum of difficulty for the attendant." In short, the focus is on not causing trouble, and as observed with American prisoners of war by Strassman, Thaler, and Schein (1956) apathy, uninvolved indifference ("playing it cool") was a reaction to and defense against the stressful situation.

Discussing the patient role, Bloom (1963, p. 191) writes that, "He is taught, first of all, *how to behave* in his new role as a hospital patient." Bloom (1963, p. 191) also notes the differences in evaluation of the same behavioral changes:

> What Beers describes as therapeutic progress, however, was not so interpreted by the staff of the several hospitals in which he was a patient. Rather, his change from a stuporous but quiet patient into an articulate, energetic, and assertive one was interpreted as an increase of disturbance. Similar experiences are described by virtually all the published autobiographical patient writings.

Dunham and Weinberg elaborate this point (pp. 123–8):

> Adherence to the routine means protection; deviation involves risks and penalties. New experiences and new events are a source of interest and excitement; but any impending change beyond their control arouses insecurities and apprehensions. . . . Length of stay itself has a positive value by making the outside community recede in the distance. . . . One factor is the patient's skewed sense of time. On the one hand, the hospital monotony leaves a "sameness" that stirs few feelings. On the other hand, the patient's few emotional experiences are so vividly recalled that they seem to have a continual recency. . . . The norm of behavior is to "get along" and to make the most of hospital facilities. In this way, the patients can obtain the tranquility necessary to make the hospital "livable." Whether consciously or unconsciously, they become oriented to hospital adjustment as an *end in itself* as the prospects of discharge become progressively dimmer and the outside world increasingly remote. They differ from hopeful patients whose hospital adjustment is merely a *means to discharge* and are oriented toward the outside world.

We should note, however, that the use of response contingent reinforcement, *if used for the benefit of the patient*, is one of the most effective forms of rehabilitation (Ullmann and Krasner, 1965). We should also indicate that strong avoidance of punishment in schizophrenics is a phenomenon that has been frequently observed in experiments making use of learning procedures (Atkinson and Robinson, 1961; McCarthy, 1964). To quote Dunham and Weinberg (p. 66): " 'Everything here is definite,' said one patient. 'You soon learn what you should do and mainly what you should not do.' "

The effects of changes from the environmental conditions of moral treatment to large, public hospitals following a medical model have been cited in this section. Perhaps the best single summary of the foregoing material was provided by Ozarin (1954) who commented, "After visiting some 35 mental hospitals, the writer has formed strong convictions that much of the pathological behavior of patients is a result of their hospital experience rather than a manifestation of their mental illness."

## THE SOCIOPSYCHOLOGICAL MODEL

In the medical model it is presumed that there is some underlying conflict, disorder, disease, or reaction to the environment which is a deviation from a normal state and must be treated prior to and as a necessary condition for altered behavior. In the field of psychiatry, the most direct effect of this analogy to physical medicine is the hypothesis of symptom substitution (Yates, 1958; Ullmann and Krasner, 1965, pp. 6–8, 13–15). A sociopsychological model argues that there is no difference between normal and abnormal behavior and that both are developed, maintained, and changed by the same principles.

A sociopsychological model deals with overt behavior in a social context. Parsons (1957) offers the following definition: "A mentally ill person is then, in my view, a person who by definition cannot get along with his fellows, who presents a problem to them directly on the behavioral level." We may note with Szasz (1963) and Ferster (1965) that a person comes to a psychiatric hospital because someone who is powerful enough to have his way, wants to change the patient. That person may be the patient himself, his relatives, employer, or the police.

The regularities which lead to diagnoses of schizophrenia are less than perfectly clear. For example Jackson (1960, p. 11) writes: "The term 'schizophrenic' in medical circles carries almost as much of a ring of authenticity as 'diabetic' or 'tubercular.' Yet it is actually nearly as much a fiction as that lovely legal appellation a 'reasonable man.' " A similar view is presented by Menninger (1959, p. 517).

> Indeed, I have tried to eliminate from my own vocabulary quite a number of words which suggest that schizophrenia *is* a disease, a disease which is also a psychosis. Now I not only believe that no such disease as schizophrenia can be clearly defined or identified or proved to exist, but I also hold that there is no such thing as a psychosis or a neurosis. My point is that no one can satisfactorily define these terms in a way which the rest of us can accept so that if we use the terms we involve ourselves in confusion because we are all, or nearly all, talking about different things. It is like a Russian, a South African, a Swiss, an American, and a South Sea Islander talking about freedom. . . . We are not all using different words for the same thing, but we are using the same words for different things.

Studies by Zigler and Phillips (1961), Wittenborn, Holzberg, and Simon (1953), and Freudenberg and Robertson (1956) are examples of evidence that the relationship between symptoms and diagnostic category is generally small and membership in a particular diagnostic group provides minimal information about the patient, especially since patients with similar symptoms may be assigned different labels, while patients with similar labels may manifest decidedly different symptom pictures. Schmidt and Fonda (1956) indicate that there is considerable disagreement among professionals about the placement of individuals in broad categories such as brain injured, psychotic, or personality disorder, and that within each of these broad categories there is increasingly frequent disagreement among the experts as to the sub-category in which the individual belongs. Further evidence on the difficulties of psychiatric diagnosis is presented by Babigian *et al.* (1965), Beck *et al.* (1962), Sandifer, Pettus, and Quade (1964), and Stoller and Geertsma (1963).

Pasamanick, Dinitz, and Lefton (1959) in discussing their data make the point very clearly:

> ... despite protestations that their point of reference is always the individual patient, clinicians in fact may be so committed to a particular school of thought, that the patient's diagnosis and treatment is largely predetermined. Clinicians, as indicated by these data, may be selectively perceiving and emphasizing only those characteristics and attributes of their patients which are relevant to their own preconceived systems of thought. As a consequence, they may be overlooking other patient characteristics which would be considered crucial by colleagues who are otherwise committed. This makes it possible for one psychiatrist to diagnose nearly all of his patients as schizophrenic while an equally competent clinician diagnoses a comparable group of patients as psychoneurotics.

The task of the diagnostician is to make a societal or administrative decision, admission to the hospital (see Mishler and Waxler, 1963), and buttress it as a medical one. Lehrman (1961) gives strong indication of the behavior influence pressures the interviewer can bring to bear as he seeks a medical justification for the legal decision of commitment. Szasz (1963) has done more than any other author in documenting and thinking through the societal implications of this situation. Our present interest in the matter is on many levels. There is the empirical problem of the role of diagnostic composition in the collection of data. There is the matter of appropriateness of treatment in terms of what is treated, that is the formulation of what effective treatment might be and the conditions which foster or hinder it. If we take the view that functional psychoses are learned behaviors and are developed, maintained, and changed by the same principles as all other learned behavior, large hospitals may be studied as social learning situations. In the previous section we saw that such hospitals may be inappropriate for effective treatment and may even be a major factor in the development and maintenance of severe maladaptive behaviors.

The medical model, manifested by Kraepelinean categorization is of a disease, an insult to the organism of a metabolic or neurological nature, which leads to the development of maladaptive behavior in the same manner that an infection, among other causes, may lead to the development of a fever. Examples of psychologists discussing abnormal behavior from the standpoint of a medical model may be found in Thorpe and Katz (1948, pp. 161–2), Hutt and Gibby (1957, pp. 78–9), and Coleman (1956, p. 225). If this model is followed, then recovery from psychosis must be based on an *indirect* treatment, one in which the cause is dealt with rather than the overt behavior which is but an indication of the presence of the cause. The current formulation of the American Psychiatric Association (1952) incorporates this model within a Freudian view of personality. For example (p. 12): "... a psychotic reaction may be defined as one in which the personality, in its struggle for adjustment to internal and external stresses, utilizes severe affective disturbances, profound autism and withdrawal from reality, and/or formation of delusions or hallucinations." The abnormal conditions, stresses, have an effect on an intervening variable, the personality, which is reified so that it "struggles" and "utilizes" severe maladaptive behavior. The treatment by either medication or insight is aimed at the personality and not at the symptomatic behavior it "utilizes."

Maladaptive behavior may be formulated, as it was during the period of moral treatment, as unique to each individual. What is added by sociopsychological formulations is that the behavior is the natural, lawful outcome of specific reinforcing contingencies which the individual has experienced in the past and which continue in the present. It should be kept in mind that the behavior of professional personnel, such as admitting psychiatrists, is influenced and shaped by the same principles of learning as patients. Treatment personnel are reinforced for selected, visible behaviors. In broad outline the behavior of both patients and treatment personnel may be said to be institutionalized, if we use the word to mean the person behaves in the manner expected of one who holds a particular social position (Balint, 1957; Bloom, 1963; Jaco, 1958; King, 1962; Levinson and Gallagher, 1964; Parsons, 1951; Ruesch, 1950). The expected behavior is confirmatory of a reinforceable pattern and reduces the difficulties or maximizes the likelihood of reinforcement of the other people with whom the employee works, and therefore eventually of himself. Examples of the variety of situations and behaviors which illustrate these principles are presented in Krasner and Ullmann (1965) and include modeling and hypnosis as well as the development and alteration of specific patterns of behavior. Jerome Frank (1961) has shown the thread of expectation and role learning from primitive and religious forms of treatment through more widely used methods of psychotherapy. Orne (1962) and Rosenthal (1963) have indicated the importance of demand characteristics, the cues indicating expected behavior, in psychological research, while Orne and

Scheibe (1964) have offered a demonstration of this point with sensory deprivation and Schachter and Singer (1962) with drugs. At a different level, there have been numerous reports of the effects of experimental manipulation of attention, interest, and pleasure on the increase or decrease of modal schizophrenic symptoms such as the expression of affect (Salzinger and Pisoni, 1958; Weiss, Krasner, and Ullmann, 1963), "sick" and "healthy" talk (Ullmann *et al.*, 1965), and delusions (Rickard, Digman, and Horner, 1960; Rickard and Dinoff, 1962). Effects of experimental operant conditioning have been noted on social behavior (King, Armitage, and Tilton, 1960; Ullmann, Krasner, and Collins, 1961) and perceptual defense (Ullmann, Weiss, and Krasner, 1963). Finally, work such as that by Ayllon (1963), Ayllon and Haughton (1964), Ayllon and Michael (1959), and Ayllon and Azrin (1965), illustrates the application of these principles in clinical situations.

Because this view differs from the generally accepted pattern of Kraepelinean diagnosis, it is possible to ask whether the regularities of diagnosis are accountable on this basis. We may remark, first, that these regularities, as pointed out by authors such as Zigler and Phillips (1961) and Wittenborn, Holzberg, and Simon (1953), are far less frequent than is usually supposed. Second, we may point out that schizophrenia is a relatively peculiar "illness" in that rapid and florid symptomatic onset is a favorable prognostic sign, and that patterns of symptoms show dramatic changes over time and place. Third, we may note that some of the most crucial symptomatic features have not been found upon careful, systematic observation (e.g. Zimet and Brackbill, 1956; Ullmann and Hunrichs, 1958). We may add that studies such as those of Binder (1956), and McGaughran and Moran (1956), fail to find a differential decrement in reasoning or concept formation, but rather a generalized social deficit and avoidance of involvement with the situation. Further, concept formation or abstract thinking may be viewed as an attainment (Becker, 1956; Werner, 1948) which through failure of environmental stimulation and support (Hayes, 1962; Hunt, 1961) may not be manifested because of a deficit in training rather than a loss through disease. We may also note that performance on abstractions (Kaufman, 1964; Meichenbaum, 1965) and common associations (Sommer, Witney, and Osmond, 1962; Ullmann, Krasner, and Edinger, 1964) may be affected directly by differential situational characteristics. Finally, theoretical explanations of how a situation may alter the likelihood of abstract responses are offered by Bridger (1964) and McReynolds (1960). The "massive affect" of Bridger and the "incongruent percepts" of McReynolds may well be heightened by the novel, threatening situation of hospital admission in which normal modes of reinforcement differ from the reinforced patient role. To obtain release the patient must do what is expected of him just as much as a person who is exposed to other forms of coercive persuasion (Schein, Schneier, and Barker, 1961). Patients must arrive at a formulation of themselves which is not only consistent with that of their physicians, but they must convince the physicians of their personal, spontaneous belief in this formulation. Whether this state may be called a confession or insight into illness (see Frank, 1961, chapter 7, for a particularly good discussion of this point), it is a "solution" to the problem of current institutional adjustment. Loeb (1957) indicates how fitting the expected pattern is rewarding for both the patient and the therapist:

> However, the patient, too, can modify this role by participating in the diagnostic culture. If he can talk about himself, his fellow patients, and the staff in terms of their "individual dynamics" he is thought to be an especially good patient, he shows insight, and he tends to get along well. In other words the therapist can relate to him in a way that goes beyond the superordination–subordination relationship involved in the doctor–mental patient dyad. They can interact as individuals.

In dealing with the behaviors of patients and staff in the environment of the large psychiatric hospital we shall use social reinforcement theory and concepts drawn from the study of learning. By learning we mean the acquisition of a functional connection between an environmental stimulus and some subject response. A stimulus which initially had no particular relevance may elicit, maintain, or increase the emission of certain responses if it has been associated with meaningful stimuli to which the organism responds.

Learned responses may generalize and be made to stimuli similar to the originally learned one. Discrimination is brought about by selective reinforcement of one of two stimuli similar to each other, and extinction of the other. The reinforced stimulus and response to it will continue to be associated with a change in the organism's behavior, while the extinguished response will decrease in frequency of emission. Withdrawal of an aversive condition is positively reinforcing and will increase the likelihood of a particular response being made in future similar situations, while cessation of a positive reinforcer is likely to be a negative reinforcer and suppress behavior on which it is contingent. Any stimulus that marks a time or place for reinforcement, positive or negative, is a discriminative stimulus. Discriminative stimuli may themselves become reinforcing, and in adult life discriminative stimuli such as money, attention, and praise, are widely effective. These concepts, positive and negative reinforcement, extinction, discrimination, generalization, and discriminative stimuli, have been reviewed here with barbaric speed. The reader who wishes a longer, more careful, and more accurate coverage is referred to textbooks of learning such as Hilgard (1956). Discussions of pathology and treatment from this viewpoint are provided by Ferster (1958, 1965), Skinner (1953), and Ullmann and Krasner (1965).

Given the foregoing material as background, it is possible to state the sociopsychological model more concisely. The phrase "socio-" is used for a number of reasons. The first is that the focus is on behavior which occurs in a social situation and is socially meaningful (Skinner, 1953, pp. 297–312). Second, the present formulation is an extension of the concepts of deviance provided by sociologists, most notably, Becker (1963). "Deviance" is not a quality of the act the person commits or a characteristic (disease) of the person himself, but the application by others of sanctions for an act which was unexpected and upsetting. The label of deviance or schizophrenia is as much a function of responses to a type of behavior as it is a function of a particular pattern of behavior emitted by the "schizophrenic." The labeller obtains his power to label and his patterns of diagnosis in a social context, and the act of calling someone a schizophrenic is as much a proper subject for sociology and psychology as the act of behaving in a schizophrenic manner. The phrase "psychological" is added to the title of this model because the social reinforcement concepts developed by psychologists provide a verifiable method for describing the variables involved in the development and categorization of deviant behavior.

We have previously in this chapter cited Miller (1957) how an increase in items leads to categorization and reaction to all members of the sub-group in a uniform, stereotyped fashion. Designation of a person as a deviant on the basis of a single characteristic or action follows this pattern. The person is reacted to as a criminal or schizophrenic: he is responded to as if he manifested all the behavior informally assigned to one so designated. This may lead to his exclusion from normal avenues of reinforcement such as employment. It may lead to reasonable requests being ignored (extinguished) because the person is a "schizophrenic." Both the patient and the staff member develop a set of expectations about what the world is like and how to deal with it and a set of routine activities based on this "assumptive" world. We may say that a deviant learns a "career" or we may say he learns to be a schizophrenic. In both instances the social environment is critically involved.

Given the orientation of a sociopsychological model, the therapeutic task of the hospital is re-education. In its broadest aspects the procedure is identical with that of the development of any pattern of behavior, whether socially sanctioned or not. The behavior currently emitted, if it is objectionable, is extinguished and possibly even made mildly aversive through treatment as a barrier to reinforcement gained by other, more socially acceptable means. The crucial factor however is that there be behavior which when emitted will be reinforced. Such behavior involves acts which are acceptable and plausible in the extra-hospital community and which are contradictory to deviant behavior. The patient must be shaped into a career of normality and find the extra-hospital culture rewarding. This implies that acts necessary outside the hospital be possible within the hospital. Next, when such acts are made, they should elicit a change in the environment. This suggests that reinforcing stimuli be made available to the hospital staff. Illustrations of such programs have been provided by Ayllon and Azrin (1965) and Atthowe and Krasner (1965). The patient can earn tokens (even as "normal" people earn money) which permit the purchase of the good things in life. Involved in such a procedure is clarity of the goal to be obtained (improved behavior, eventual discharge) and an explicit method.

There is an ethical implication to this viewpoint which must be made explicit. If schizophrenia is a disease, then it is a deviation from optimum functioning and it is legitimate to treat it by any and all professional means (shock, drugs, surgery, psychoanalytic psychotherapy, social reinforcement procedures) currently available. The presence of abnormality justifies the treatment. However, if the behavior that categorizes a person as schizophrenic is deviant only as a function of the responses of others to it and is, at the level of learning, essentially normal, then the person who labels and treats is faced with a new ethical problem. His treatment will involve the creation of the conditions under which people are likely to become members of new groups (Toch, 1965), or, from their starting point, "outsiders" (Becker, 1963). The therapist, just as the supervisor and administrator, assumes the responsibility for manipulating the environment in a manner likely to increase certain behaviors and decrease others. In short, there is overt behavior influence. An employee or a voluntary patient may be conceived of as having made a contract and having the choice to terminate the association. The committed patient cannot be conceived in this manner. His detection, incarceration, and treatment, if he is not considered to be suffering from an illness, is similar to that of a criminal. We consider society's treatment of criminals to be legitimate because no one has a right to break laws. However, due to our training within a medical model and the dangers inherent in the conflict between civil liberties and loose definitions of inappropriate social behavior, we are loathe to accept the analogy between the criminal and the psychotic. Although current psychiatric practice may at times already define mental illness so broadly as to endanger civil liberties in some cases, the sociopsychological model makes the problem of responsibility explicit.

## WHAT SHOULD THE HOSPITAL ACCOMPLISH?

As was implicit in the previous sections of this chapter, and as explicitly argued by Strauss *et al.* (1964, pp. 359 et seq.) ideology affects the type and organization of treatment and different ideological convictions generate their own morality. The behaviors which will be encouraged in a given hospital vary with the frame of reference of its staff. A dynamically oriented hospital will differ radically from a custodial one. Strauss *et al.* (1964) document this assertion in detail. A flavor of the problem of differing ideologies may be obtained by a tongue-in-cheek statement by Cohen (1957) about a patient's seemingly "spontaneous" improvement: "This brought me no cheer since it appeared that he might make a social recovery without ever analyzing his conflicts, which, in this hospital at that time, was considered a fate next to life-long illness." The orientations of moral treatment, the medical model of the late nineteenth century, current psychoanalytically oriented ego-psychology (for an outstanding example, see Cumming and Cumming, 1962), and behavioristic sociopsychological theory would lead to specification of considerably different modes of staff behavior as desirable.

We would like to argue that the goal of all techniques are similar to the extent of viewing discharge as of some positive social value. Parsons (1957) writes that the criterion of discharge is the cessation of the need to be hospitalized. There is however the problem of the difference between the hospital and the outside community in defining this need. Schwartz and Schwartz (1964, p. 147) note that required behavior in the institution is often inappropriate and sometimes even contradictory to the requirements of the normal adult world. The hospital staff may well have to decide the point at which the patient has achieved a point of diminishing returns such that gains in terms of the alleviation of residual psychiatric symptoms are more than negated by the process of disculturation associated with prolonged hospitalization. Another conflict among ideologies is whether deviant behavior should be "accepted" (for example, Hyde and Williams, 1957) or extinguished (for example, Ayllon and Michael, 1959; Atthowe and Krasner, 1965).

This problem is reflected in the very foundations of the present study. While it was possible to find empirical evidence to support the hypothesis that increasing size would be negatively associated with effectiveness, no similar body of evidence could be obtained for increasing staff per patient. Rather, the literature is replete with numerous and frequently conflicting reports of how staff might best be used. The literature reflects the correct procedure: it is not important how many people work at a hospital but what they do. Hoffman (1957) states this neatly when he writes: "To a limited extent, one can achieve the effect of increased numbers of personnel by learning to utilize more effectively the existing personnel."

Endeavoring to be as general as possible, we may posit that a first requirement is simply staff contact with patients and a second requirement is that such contact be with a person oriented toward the return of the patient to his community. The first requirement leads directly to a hypothesis that increased numbers of staff per patient will be positively associated with increased effectiveness because, by chance, there will be increased staff-patient contact. It is also consistent with material reviewed in the previous chapter: smaller hospitals should have greater staff participation and therefore be more effective.

This first requirement makes no statement as to what the participating staff member should do. It is perhaps analogous to saying that for therapy to take place there must be a therapist. It states neither the goals nor the methods of treatment, but rather, other things being equal, human contact in the large public psychiatric hospital is likely to be beneficial. In an outstandingly hard-headed look at psychiatric hospitals Perrow (1965) argues that many of the difficulties which have been blamed on poor communication and ineffective organization are more reasonably ascribed to the lack of an effective technology for treating psychiatric patients. Because Perrow is in many respects the most incisive critic of the position taken in this book, his work is of particular value. Perrow (1965, p. 934) notes that "Too many of the structural changes announced in the literature have produced no lasting results; too many of the results appear to be due to the 'Hawthorne' effect, whereby merely to show some interest in patients and to increase interaction has a beneficial effect—although it may disappear as soon as the research team or change agents leave the scene." In a later section Perrow (1965, p. 941) writes: "There is a persistent theme in the literature that almost anything can have its effect where conditions are bad. Kamman and his associates reported on a survey of 90 articles on psychotherapy with schizophrenics. They found a wide variation in technique, theory, and qualifications of the therapists and concluded that 'almost anything that has at one time or another been tried has been of benefit in the treatment of schizophrenia' (Kamman *et al.*, 1954)." Finally, Perrow (1965, p. 942) quotes Glass (1957, p. 526) to the effect that possibly, ". . . milieu therapy is another way in which enthusiasm is communicated by the treatment personnel, and this is the crucial factor in the treatment. . . ." This argument may be extended to the administration of tranquilizing drugs:

> It is undoubtedly true that some proportion of the improvement from the drugs is due to the increased interest and attention of the hospital personnel. The double-blind studies have all indicated that 20–30% of the placebo-treated patients show some degree of improvement. . . . Another advantage of the drug treatment is the elevation of morale of the hospital personnel, especially those dealing with chronic patients. There is definitely less of a hopeless attitude toward such patients, and the greater interaction between the patient and the personnel is undoubtedly a pronounced factor in contributing to the lesser tension of the patients. It may well be that this is the most important benefit of the drugs. . . . (Freeman, 1958, p. 499.)

Observations of this type have led authors such as Frank (1961),

Goldstein (1962), and Stotland and Kobler (1965) to place great emphasis on patient–therapist expectancies or simply the generation of hope.

The finding of the wide range of techniques which have measurable benefit and the positive effect of methods which are so non-specific as to be placebos is one of the strongest arguments for a formulation of schizophrenic reaction as a sociopsychological phenomenon rather than a biophysical illness. The impact of a placebo is along psychological dimensions rather than directly physiological ones. It is probably for this reason that despite its almost central place in the history of medicine (Shapiro, 1960; Honigfeld, 1963; U.S. Department of Health, Education, and Welfare, 1963) the person who responds favorably to a placebo is looked upon with disfavor: he was not *really* sick. In similar fashion, when a person remarks that the improvement was a "Hawthorne" or placebo effect, he overlooks the improvement itself just as much as if he overlooked the increased items manufactured during the time of the experimental manipulation called the "Hawthorne" effect. Given the view that schizophrenic reaction is a sociopsychological phenomenon, and given the beneficial effect of non-specific therapy, it seems reasonable for the uppermost administrative levels to seek out and encourage situations which lead to increased instances of staff interaction with patients. The technology of the administrator may be in large measure the generation and maintenance of "Hawthorne" effects.

However, it would be wrong to state that all staff-patient interactions are equally beneficial. This leads to the second general requirement, that the staff person should be oriented toward the return of the patient to his community. This requirement is general enough to win a wide range of acceptance. This requirement, however, entails a number of implicit assumptions which deserve amplification. The expectations of the staff have an effect on the frequency and manner of interaction with patients. A clear statement of this point is offered by Cumming and Cumming (1957, pp. 68–9):

> It is assumed that the patient will neither leave the hospital nor be eligible for an equalitarian relationship with the staff member. When under the conditions of overcrowding outlined above, a promising candidate is sought for discharge, the stable caste relationship on the ward is interrupted and a new type of relationship emerges. If a patient is considered for discharge, an implicit hypothesis about him is formed among the staff members: "This person is able to carry on an acceptable social life in the outside world." One way of testing this hypothesis is to interact with this person as if he were a normal individual and to notice

how he responds. . . . What starts as an experiment has unintended consequences. The staff member's initiation of normal social interaction brings into play a whole network of expectations which often bring the patient into closer conformity with socially acceptable conduct.

Kennard (1957) reports a similar finding. Due to remodeling, there were shifts in the locale of both patients and staff and a resultant change in the disposition of patients. Kennard writes, "The conclusion seems inescapable that the difference in results is not due to the current psychiatric condition of the patient, but is due to the presence of the staff which is able to sift through the patients and work with those who were accessible to existing forms of therapy."

A final illustration of administrative changes on patient discharge involves two fascinating papers by Reimanis (1965a, 1965b). In January, 1965, plans to close a number of Veterans Administration institutions were announced. Reimanis found that at his installation anomie increased significantly in both patients and staff, but that furloughs and regular discharges also increased significantly.

In preparing the patient for return to *the* community, it is important that the focus be the return of the patient to *his* community. The range of values and appropriate behaviors sought should be in reference to the patient's sub-group and not the psychiatrist's. The preceding quotations as well as the data cited in the first chapter would make us hesitant over the importance of "personality integration." Similarly, it is reasonable to ask whether the professional staff does not do a disservice when it focuses on "insight" rather than behavioral change. Insight may be a reasonable criterion for outpatient treatment or for a person in a professional sub-group, but it may be an irrelevant variable for the majority of sub-groups which comprise the general population. Finally, it may well be that changed behavior precedes rather than follows changes in intra-psychic dynamics: being different may permit the patient to evaluate his former behavior in the light of his current behavior.

The second requirement essentially involves the first (interaction) with the added stipulation of the goal (return of the patient to his extra-hospital community). A third requirement would involve the methods by which this goal might be most expeditiously achieved. If schizophrenic reaction is essentially a sociopsychological phenomenon rather than a biophysical illness, and if, as has been argued, psychological variables rather than physiological ones are the most relevant ones to manipulate, then the emphasis would shift from treatment in a physician-patient model to re-education in a teacher-student model. Under this condition, it might be hypothesized that the systematic application of learning principles and the findings of experiments on behavior influence (Krasner and Ullmann, 1965) would lead to effective and efficient behavioral change. In addition to the material presented by Ullmann and Krasner (1965), Paul (1964) and Davison (1965) have provided experimental evidence for such a contention. This third requirement will not be further pursued at this point because other than a few scattered experiments (Peters and Jenkins, 1954; King, Armitage, and Tilton, 1960), direct application of learning procedures had not had wide use or major impact in VA hospitals at the time of the present study.

## SUMMARY

In this chapter we have reviewed a number of historical and theoretical issues. We remarked on the success of the moral treatment of the insane in the first half of the nineteenth century. We then noted the changes associated with the decline of moral treatment and the rise of large, public psychiatric hospitals following a medical model and involving an aide culture. In so doing, we cited reports descriptive of the majority of wards in large psychiatric hospitals. Finally, we introduced a sociopsychological model and set forth two very general requirements or goals for the hospital staff. The first requirement was staff contact with patients and the second requirement was that the staff person interacting with the patient be oriented toward the patient's return to his community. These two general requirements for staff behavior were related to the major hypotheses of the present research on effectiveness of psychiatric hospitals. Specific professions and behaviors were not touched on; these will be discussed after analysis of data has provided us with differential correlations between types of staffing and measures of effectiveness.

## CHAPTER 4

# *Studies Comparing Hospitals*

WITH the exception of work by Jones and Sidebotham (1962) and the Veterans Administration's Psychiatric Evaluation Project, there is a relative paucity of quantitative material systematically comparing the effectiveness of different psychiatric hospitals. In this chapter, after briefly mentioning some of the other available literature, we shall devote separate sections to reviewing these two studies.

Strauss *et al.* (1964) contrast a psychoanalytically oriented psychiatric ward within a general medical setting with a state mental hospital. The multitude of differences between the two organizations do not permit isolation or statistical analysis of single variables. Highly suggestive data were reported by Hess, Riedel, and Fitzpatrick (1961, p. 69) as a by-product of their development of a model sample of general medical (rather than psychiatric) hospitals. The upper ranges of number of discharges per hospital bed were as follows: 500 or more beds, 42; 250–499 beds, 59; 100–249 beds, 61; 50–99 beds, 61; under 50 beds, 74. The type of patients admitted to different hospitals and the pressures for turnover (for example, in the under-50-bed hospital group the low ratios occurred in populous urban areas and the highest ratios in the small community hospitals), are variables which must be taken into account. The trend of the data, however, is consistent with the hypothesis that small size is associated with favorable effects.

A quantitative approach to comparisons of the milieu of hospitals is made possible by the work of Jackson (1964). Jackson collected comparative data on four large mental hospitals within a state system. His instrument was the CTE, Characteristics of the Treatment Environment. The CTE asks whether the hospital environment provides the patient with opportunities to practice and learn behaviors which are considered adjustive in the extra-hospital community. Jackson draws heavily on the Sullivanian tradition, and particularly the work of Schwartz (1957) to select areas of behavior.

Relevant personnel rate the frequency of situations which indicate patients' initiative, increasing patients' self-esteem, reducing patients' anxiety, helping patients understand their illness, reducing patients' distortions of reality, and increasing patients' social participation. The items deal with the frequency of various patient activities and privileges, frequency of certain staff interactions, and hospital policies such as the "open door." In short, staff observers are used to measure the frequency of behaviors and policies by which the treatment milieu may be operationally defined. In Jackson's (1964) work the CTE was sensitive to differences between hospitals, continued and intensive treatment units, and different staff elements.

A study similar to that of Jones and Sidebotham was conducted on a pilot group of three hospitals by Wadsworth, Tonge, and Barber (1957). After adding the cost of lost earnings, these authors concluded that the hospital with the highest cost per patient-week had the lowest cost per case because of the rapidity with which patients were restored to the community.

Wing and Brown (1961) also studied three English mental hospitals. Their interest was in variables such as amount of personal freedom, clinical disturbance, and nurses' optimism, rather than discharge, size, or staffing of the hospitals. The findings were in general supportive of the concepts of the therapeutic community.

Data concerning the association between hospital characteristics such as size and staffing and measures of effectiveness such as release rates were computed from data presented by Bockoven (1963, fig. 1, p. 23, table 3, p. 28, and fig. 3, p. 56). For data concerning the operation of Worcester State Hospital over twelve consecutive decades, rank-order correlations were .76 ($p < .01$) between per cent of admissions released and physicians per patient, and −.89 ($p < .001$) between per cent of admissions released and the size of the patient population.

## THE WORK OF JONES AND SIDEBOTHAM

Jones and Sidebotham (1962) surveyed three English mental hospitals. One of these hospitals was a 300-bed private institution, Crown Lodge, which provided care and treatment of an unusually high standard for a privileged group of patients. As an independent hospital, Crown Lodge had some advantages over Health Service hospitals: there was the spur of the necessity for survival, which meant ready adaptation to changing conditions; swift decision-making, because decisions were the responsibility of a small group and did not have to be referred to a higher level; and a capacity for experimentation, typified in the "therapeutic community" which few Health Service hospitals possessed.

An insight into the personal care found in a small hospital is given when Jones and Sidebotham note that the files were disorganized and it was difficult to gather follow-up material from them. They write (p. 47): "but the hospital is so small, and the service to patients so individual, that members of staff had little difficulty in recalling from memory the salient facts about any particular patient." This may be contrasted with the situation in Belknap's large, state hospital in which the psychiatrists spent a majority of their time in administrative and report-writing tasks, tasks which were unpleasant and unprofessional and which may have added to the staff turnover. Belknap (1956, p. 246) quotes the superintendent: "If they ever stayed", he said, "they could keep most of it in their heads."

A second hospital discussed by Jones and Sidebotham is Moordale, a small, 400-bed hospital which, for financial reasons, became affiliated with the Health Service. To quote Jones and Sidebotham (1962, p. 104): "Because it is a small hospital, and perhaps because it is in some ways threatened by group organization, it is exceptionally united." An example of difficulties with a larger, administrative unit is provided by Jones and Sidebotham (1962, p. 89) in their discussion of the problems of the Catering Officer. This man was at times sent (and charged for on the budget) items which he did not want or could not use. The lists of his requests for the hospital "are subject to alteration at hospital or group level, without prior consultation or subsequent notification. The catering officer submits his lists. In due course, he receives his supplies, less any items vetoed by his unseen mentors. He does not know the name or official position of the person who actually handles his lists at Group. . . ."

The third hospital, Northtown, seems a typical large public psychiatric hospital. Jones and Sidebotham (1962, p. 63) write:

> . . . there are 2750 patients in the hospital. Of these, nearly 1000 are on closed wards, many of them of the old asylum type. In all, there are probably not more than 450 or 500 short-stay patients at any one time, as against more than 2000 long-stay. The discharge rate for 1958 was 97%, which is high; but this means that a small proportion of short-stay beds turned over several times, while the great bulk of the hospital population was unchanged.

Jones and Sidebotham describe various instances at Northtown of poor communication which were relatable to large size. Jones and Sidebotham (p. 77) describe the situation as follows:

> Most members of staff were reasonably well-informed about members of their own professional group—provided they worked in the same part of the hospital; and we formed a strong impression of a series of almost water-tight groups, working side by side, but making very little impact on one another. Doctors, nurses and administrators belong to large and well-organized professional groups, and do not feel a lack of communication, because they tend to think primarily within the professional orbit; but members of smaller groups and newer professions, such as the psychologists, the social workers, and others, are very dependent on cooperation with other groups, and do not always secure it.

In their description of turnover in the large (Northtown) hospital, Jones and Sidebotham make the point that this turnover was found with recent admissions. To continue with this point, because it is vital to the need for two measures of effectiveness (Jones and Sidebotham, 1962, p. 142): "The overwhelming majority of patients discharged are voluntary patients, although each hospital has in the standing population a fair proportion of certified patients (Crown Lodge 27.6 per cent, Moordale 23.3 per cent. Northtown has a very high proportion, 79.8 per cent). This confirms the picture of each hospital as 'two hospitals'—one large static, and the other with a rapid turnover."

Jones and Sidebotham's work with samples of discharged patients confirms the very low probability that after two years, a patient will be discharged. Finally, in their tables 25 and 28 (pp. 168 and 170, respectively) it is made clear that the long-stay patient receives less treatment as measured by cost per week. While at the small private hospital nursing care and drug costs may be slightly greater for long-stay patients than short-care patients, this was not true for the other two hospitals. In all three hospitals, more medical effort was invested in the short-stay than long-stay patients, the ratio of costs being approximately four times greater for short-stay than for long-stay patients.

Jones and Sidebotham (1962) make a serious and scholarly attempt to devise a measure of efficiency, a measure of cost per successful product. (The present work will deal with the more modest goal of a measure of effectiveness, the frequency with which the desired product is attained.) Two difficulties arise. The first is the problem of a correction for readmission. Jones and Sidebotham (1962, p. 125) point out that "The moment of discharge is not a suitable one for making a judgment on the patient's condition; for he is about to leave a known environment, in which his reactions have been observed, for the unknown stresses of life in the community. Whether he does in fact recover may depend more on what the community at large does to him than on what the hospital has done for him."

The differences in the relapse rates of the three hospitals studied by Jones and Sidebotham were so slight that no statistical significance was attached to them and the probability of relapse was treated as a constant. The problem of a correction for relapse then becomes academic.

The second problem was that Jones and Sidebotham restricted their efforts to short-stay, first admissions. That is, all the patients in the sample on which they computed efficiency left the hospital within two years. Jones and Sidebotham (1962, p. 172) remark that at one end of this time period are the very short-stay patients: "A few patients discharge themselves after two or three days in hospital, and there is a good case for disregarding those whose length of stay is less than a fortnight on the grounds that they have not been in the hospital long enough to receive active treatment." (In the present work, a minimum of seven days was set to rule out such instances as well as administrative or "paper" admissions. However, the present research agreed with Jones and Sidebotham: this extra precaution makes little difference when the sample includes 100 or more patients.)

Jones and Sidebotham ruled out patients whose stay had been longer than two years. Given the small chances of a discharge after two years of hospitalization, this procedure also did not influence appreciably their final results. The effect of this maneuver, however, is that the efficiency measure was limited to the group with which the hospital was effective. It is cost per success based on successes only and does not take into account what per cent of admissions did eventually become successes. Because the admissions and discharges compared to resident population were far greater, and because the hospitals were smaller and more highly staffed, it is reasonable to presume that Crown Lodge and Moordale had a higher percentage of successes than Northtown. If the cost of failures, patients not discharged, were included into the efficiency measure as an "overhead" factor, there would probably be an increase in the differences among hospitals reported by Jones and Sidebotham.

Jones and Sidebotham found that the cost per case was lowest in the more expensive private hospital. The average length of stay in days for the samples was 69.3 for Crown Lodge, 102.0 for Moordale, and 116.8 for Northtown. While size and staff per patient are difficult to separate in this study, the results provide empirical support for the hypotheses that small size and high staff are associated with favorable results.

## THE WORK OF THE PSYCHIATRIC EVALUATION PROJECT (PEP)

As mentioned in the preface, the immediate precursor of the present work was a project in which 12 VA hospitals were studied. The following summary will draw on the three preliminary reports of the project which are in the general literature, papers by Jenkins and Gurel (1959), Jenkins (1961), and a symposium chaired by Dr. J. J. Blasko at the 1964 convention of the American Psychological Association.

To quote Cohen (1964):

> In the main study, all patients entered the PEP (Psychiatric Evaluation Project) sample who were admitted (or more frequently readmitted) to the PEP hospitals during the year beginning August 1956, or until a quota of 120 had been reached and who met the following criteria: male, diagnosed functional psychotic, under 60, not suffering from TB or organic brain damage, and not hospitalized for more than 90 days of the 180 days prior to admission.

It should be explicit that while each hospital endeavored to meet a quota of 120 patients, some managed to complete this requirement within seven months while others continued intake over a year and attained only slightly over 50% of the number required. The final sample reported on by Cohen (1964) was composed of 1274 patients who were still alive four years after admission. Patients who had died at any time during the four-year study period, regardless of cause or date of death, were excluded from the PEP sample. Next, it should be noted that men returning to the hospitals from interruptions of hospitalization such as Trial Visits or Absences Without Leave, were admitted into the PEP sample, i.e. admissions which did not necessarily signal the start of a "new hospitalization" as defined by addition to the patients on the hospital roles.

The patients once admitted to the sample were interviewed and rated at various times within the hospital, or, if discharged, in the community through social work follow-up. To the best of the staffs' abilities there was developed a day by day record of entrance and exit into various hospitals during the four years following the admission. Such a record was probably very accurate because the patients were veterans. Every admission or discharge to a Veterans Administration hospital is routinely reported and entered in the veteran's claim folder. Further, there is a very high probability that there will be a record of an admission to a state hospital because such notification places the patient on a waiting list for transfer to a VA hospital. Contacts by project and cooperating social agencies, social workers, and routine pension examination interviews, provided further information. In short, a highly accurate, if not perfect, record of time in community and in institutions during four years was obtained.

From this material, three types of scores were developed. The first was a cross-sectional score, the patients' whereabouts at various "check points" such as 90, 180, 365 and 730 days after admission. The check points were dichotomous for the patient being "out" or "in" psychiatric or penal institutions. A second type of score was a longitudinal score of total number of Incommunity Days (ICD) during a specified period of time, e.g., 90, 180, 365, or 730 days after admission. Time in hospitals other than the one to which the patient was admitted was subtracted from incommunity days.

The third score was First Significant Release, FSR. An early FSR was defined, for purposes of the PEP study, as leaving the admitting hospital for 90 consecutive days. In the PEP study, the 24 patients who were transferred directly to another institution, whether this occurred three weeks or three years after admission, were excluded from the sample (i.e., where the ICD criterion was established for 1274 patients the FSR sample included 1250 patients). However, in the PEP study, despite the availability of scrupulous follow-up, if a man entered another hospital after having been less than 90 days in the community, as long as he did not return to his original hospital, he obtained a first significant release. Unlike the present study, no minimal time in the hospital was set; a single day was sufficient for inclusion for a four-year follow-up. The PEP study sample criteria included "functional psychotic" as the diagnostic limitation, and this meant that 95% of the sample were diagnosed schizophrenic reaction.

PEP studied 12 hospitals. Jenkins (1961) described the sample of hospitals as follows:

Twelve VA NP hospitals have been included, geographically distributed from coast to coast and varying in size from 500 beds to nearly 2000 beds. There are four new hospitals with small nursing units of the "Haun-Style" architecture. These hospitals ranged from 500 beds to 935 beds. All of these "Haun" hospitals have high staffing ratios—that is, they have more total staff than patients. There were four large old style hospitals, ranging in size from 1598 beds to 1961 beds and having low staffing ratios—more patients than staff. There were three small, old style hospitals, ranging from 652 beds to 1337 beds, also with low staffing ratios. The one old style hospital (1038 beds) with a high staffing ratio was rebuilt in a new style architecture, and the transfer from the old buildings occurred during the course of this study.

It should also be mentioned that three of the 12 hospitals devoted over one-sixth of their beds to general medical and surgical cases.

The major criterion used by the PEP study was Incommunity Days, ICD, a continuous variable making use of the maximum amount of follow-up data. Cohen (1964) notes that "although a patient may lose incommunity days either by a delayed release or a return to the hospital, most of the variance is due to delayed release."

The method of correction for potential differences among the patients admitted to different hospitals was (Cohen, 1964):

. . . an analysis of covariance with multiple covariates. Using *within*-hospital pooled correlations, we taught our computer to do multiple regression analyses, using 64 admission control variables as "predictors" against each of our release/community stay criterion variables. . . . With the regression equation we get, we plug in for each patient his standing on the 64 control variables and get our *predicted* one year ICD. This is the number of community days in the first year he is *entitled* to, given his admission characteristics. If we now subtract this from his *actual* one year ICD, the discrepancy measures among other things the effect of his hospital. . . . When this is done for all 1274 patients and the data are organized by hospital, we can see whether some hospitals have larger average values than others and to what these average differences relate.

Gurel (1964) making use of these procedures reported on the association of size (ADPL, average daily patient load) and staff–patient ratio for the 12 hospitals.

TABLE 1. (*after Gurel 1964*). *Correlations between ICD (incommunity days) and size and staffing within various times of admission at 12 hospitals*

| | 6 mos | 1 yr | 2 yr | 3 yr | 4 yr |
|---|---|---|---|---|---|
| Size | −.72 | −.70 | −.53 | −.43 | −.36 |
| Staff/patient | .59 | .53 | .44 | .37 | .30 |

With 12 cases, a correlation of .50 is significant at the .05 with one-tail test.

TABLE 2. (*after Gurel, 1964*). *Correlations between percentage of FSR (first significant release) and size and staffing obtained within various times of admission at 12 hospitals*

| | 3 mos | 6 mos | 9 mos | 1 yr | 2 yr | 3 yr |
|---|---|---|---|---|---|---|
| Size | —.68 | —.72 | —.63 | —.56 | —.18 | —.20 |
| Staff/patient | .56 | .46 | .43 | .37 | .09 | .05 |

With 12 cases, a correlation of .50 is significant at the .05 with one-tail test.

Gurel (1964) presented data on the association between size and staffing and two other criteria. The first dealt with effectiveness with chronic patients who had been transferred into PEP study hospitals after two or more years of continuous hospitalization at some other state or VA hospital. Stumpf (1964) presented the procedure and data for this study. For 11 hospitals for which data were available, size was correlated —.28 with relative effectiveness while staff–patient ratio was correlated .49. Staffing would seem to be of somewhat greater import than size with this more chronic population (with 11 cases, the .49 correlation is between the .10 and .05 levels of significance with one-tail test). A second additional criterion measure reported by Gurel (1964) deals with turnover, the number of terminated cases per size of hospital. Turnover was further broken down between total turnover and NP (neuropsychiatric) turnover. This is necessary when it is remembered that a quarter of the PEP hospitals had a major general medical mission. The correlation between size and total (including general medical) turnover was —.60 while between size and NP turnover it was —.68. The correlations were .88 between staff–patient ratio and total turnover and .57 between staff–patient ratio and psychiatric turnover.

The data presented by Gurel seem to indicate that both small size and high staffing are associated favorably with measures of effectiveness. While they form a basis for hypotheses, two major issues arise. The first is that size and staffing are not independent of each other for these 12 hospitals, and, in fact, the product-moment correlation between them was —.73. As such, for example, with the FSR measure, it is questionable whether a measure of staff–patient ratio adds anything to the results obtained by small size alone.

A second matter brought to light by Gurel's paper deals with the release criteria. Both FSR and ICD when computed at successive dates are very directly influenced by part-whole effects. With ICD, every day that is earned during the first six months is credited to the score for the first year, and every incommunity day during the first year is credited in the score for the first two years, and so forth. In similar fashion, once a person has established an early FSR within a certain period of time, he has established that date for his FSR from thence onward. Whatever percentage of early FSR is established at a hospital in the first three months is added to the early FSR percentage during the second three months, and this total is added to the percentage establishing an early FSR during the next three months, and so forth. The criteria are not independent of each other. Further, given the expectation of high positive intercorrelations among various ICD scores and various FSR measures, the steady decline in the association of both these measures with both size and staffing is a cause for concern. What is clear from graphic presentations (Gurel, 1964) is that the effects of size and staffing steadily decrease as time from admission increases. For example, following Gurel's slide 1 (1964) the difference between the four smallest and four largest hospitals was 27.7 days in the community at six months. The following six months increased this difference by 21.1 days. To the difference in ICD which existed at one year, the following (second) year added only 13.9 days, the year after that (third) 9.3 days, and the final (fourth) year 5.4 days. The matter is similar with FSR, possibly because the more men who have *not* established an FSR, the greater is the likelihood, simply by chance, that they will establish one in the future.

We have touched upon the correlation between size and staffing and noted that it was not clear, because of the significant overlap, what the effect was of size *per se*, or of staffing *per se*. We also touched on the influence of general medical cases on turnover. To determine the effects of a particular staffing pattern or treatment program it is necessary to hold certain measures constant, notably size, general medical involvement, and overall staffing. We would expect and in fact do find that as total staff increases, the vast majority of all staffing elements increase in comparison to patient population. Davis (1964) presented empirical information from a variety of factor-analytic procedures to support the necessity of this procedure, i.e., "... the first factor in any of these extractions takes out the variance associated with differential size. A second factor is also fairly obvious as a dimension associated with general medical and surgical treatment. . . ." It is only after these two factors are taken into consideration that one may properly investigate particular staffing patterns or programs. The procedure called for requires the evaluation and analysis of intercorrelations and to the extent that the PEP study did not do this, its findings raise as many questions as they answer.

## SUMMARY

In this chapter we have reviewed additional empirical studies relevant to the two major hypotheses of this study. While previous investigations do not permit the separate study of the effects of the variable of size and the variable of staffing, they do support the hypotheses that size is negatively associated with effectiveness and increased staffing is positively associated with effectiveness. The discussion of the PEP study and the work of Jones and Sidebotham also introduced a closer investigation of some of the methodological problems and strategies involved in research in this area.

With this chapter we have come to the end of our review of concepts, literature, and background. The next part of this book will present the empirical procedures and results which will be discussed in the third and final part.

# PART II

## *Procedures and Results*

# CHAPTER 5

# *Two Preliminary Studies*

A NUMBER of issues needed to be investigated prior to a test of the core hypotheses dealing with the association of measures of effectiveness with size and staffing. The method of data presentation will reflect the sequential decisions made in the present exploration. Detailed discussions of variables and decisions will be presented with the tasks in which they were involved. The first area which had to be investigated was the matter of potential differences in sampling at the various hospitals under investigation.

## CORRECTIONS FOR POTENTIAL SAMPLE DIFFERENCES

A common assumption is that differences among hospitals in their effectiveness may be the result of differences among the hospitals in the type of patients with which they work. In the present study, patients serve as items to test the "subjects," the hospitals. It is necessary that the "tests" be of equal difficulty. This need led both in the original PEP study and the present work to an investigation of patient characteristics with which to correct for differences among samples admitted to different hospitals. It should not be forgotten, however, that the procedure starts out with an assumption: that differences do in fact alter the relative standings of the hospitals. This means that not only must there be patient characteristics that are predictive of early release, but that the hospitals admit sufficiently different proportions of relatively good and poor prognostic patients *so as to change the ordering of the hospitals on the measure of effectiveness.*

### *Data obtained from hospitals*

The following material was obtained from 36 VA psychiatric hospitals: (a) a list of the names, unit numbers, and diagnoses for all admissions for two fiscal years (July 1, 1959 through June 30, 1961) and (b) a photocopy of VA Form 10–2593, Record of Hospitalization (see Appendices 1 and 2), for all schizophrenic males admitted during the first of these two years.

Use of the VA's unit (identifying) number procedure permitted a check on possible readmission to the same hospital during the entire second fiscal year. When additional material (because of transfer or readmission) was needed to determine the outcome of a case, the hospital registrars were contacted.

The VA's Record of Hospitalization form was imprinted at time of admission with 34 items of information. Of these the current research used name, identifying unit number, date of admission, date of birth, sex, marital status, and whom to notify in case of emergency. As treatment proceeded, established clinical diagnoses were entered on the form, as were all absences from the hospital. In cases where the patient received more than one diagnosis, further specification was made of which diagnosis had been responsible for the major part of the hospital stay. The form also contained material as to the final disposition of the case: discharge, transfer, or death.

The VA's Record of Hospitalization form was used to identify during a full year all males, under 60 years of age at admission, for whom a schizophrenic reaction was cited as responsible for the major part of their hospital stay. Men whose diagnoses were changed from schizophrenic reaction were dropped from the study.

### *Early release criterion, FSR*

The material from the VA Record of Hospitalization was used to determine whether each patient achieved an early or late first significant release (FSR). *An early FSR was defined as leaving the hospital within 274 calendar days of admission and remaining in the community at least 90 consecutive days.* A late FSR was defined as a failure to establish an early FSR. The number 274 was chosen as it represents the maximum number of days during a year after which a 90-day follow-up can be made. The major reason for selecting this measure was the high association between early FSR (for 90 days within 274 calendar days of admission) and other measures of release and community stay.

For 1250 patients in the PEP study, FSR within 274 calendar days had a biserial correlation of .86 with incommunity days during the first year following admission to the study.[1] In work with hospitals, however, individual patients are used as items by which to evaluate or score a hospital, and, using the PEP study data for 12 hospitals, FSR within 274 days of admission yielded product-moment correlations of .94 with total incommunity days (ICD) during the first year; .94 with ICD during two years, .94 for three years, and .93 for four years of follow-up.[2] In short, whether dealing with cases in terms of patients or cases in terms of hospitals, FSR was highly related with total incommunity days over lengthy periods of time.

Those patients for whom an unequivocal early or late FSR could not be established, due to death or transfer prior to 275 calendar days of admission, were dropped from the study. In accordance with eliminating from the study all equivocal cases, a minimum length of hospitalization, seven days, was required for inclusion in the sample and administrative or "paper" admissions were discarded. The unit number system permitted checks on readmissions and transfers and made it certain that each man was counted once only.

### *The use of marital status*

Marital status frequently has been found to be the most useful single item of information predictive of early release from psychiatric hospitals. Examples of recent studies supporting this are those by Brown (1960), Farina, Garmezy, and Barry (1963), and Johnson and McNeal (1964).

A first approach made use of all 36 hospitals. Marital status was categorized in three steps: *Marital 1* comprised married men who listed their wives as the people to notify in case of emergency; *Marital 2* comprised those men who had been married at some time during their lives but who did not list wives as the people to notify

[1] See table 3, Mimeographed Intramural Report 63–3: *Release and Community Stay Criteria in Evaluating Psychiatric Treatment*, prepared by the Psychiatric Evaluation Project, VA Hospital, Washington 7, D.C., March, 1963.

[2] See table 9, *ibid.*

in case of emergency (divorced, separated, widowed); *Marital 3* comprised those men who were single and had never married.

### *Analysis of data*

The first step was to pool the cases from all the hospitals and evaluate the association between early or late FSR and the three marital categories. Table 3 presents this material. As may be seen from Table 3, marital status and frequency of early release were highly associated, the chi-square with two degrees of freedom being 421.19. It is worth noting that marital step number 2 differed significantly from the other two categories. The chi-square values, with one degree of freedom, for the association between frequency of early release and marital steps 1 and 2 was 62.28 while the association between marital steps 2 and 3 and frequency of early release yielded a chi-square of 116.21.

TABLE 3. *The association between three types of marital status and early or late first significant release (FSR) for 8060 male schizophrenic admissions*

| | Early FSR | Late FSR | Sum | % early FSR |
|---|---|---|---|---|
| Married, wife next of kin | 1729 | 610 | 2339 | 73.9% |
| Married, wife not next of kin | 1120 | 637 | 1757 | 63.7% |
| Single, never married | 1914 | 2050 | 3964 | 48.3% |
| Sum | 4763 | 3297 | 8060 | 59.1% |

Chi-square, 2 degrees of freedom, = 421.19; $p < .001$.

The next step was to determine the association between frequency of early FSR and the three marital statuses for each of the 36 hospitals. For each hospital tables with the layout of Table 3 were developed. The obtained range of chi-squares with two degrees of freedom was from 0.00 to 28.57. The median chi-square value for 36 hospitals was 11.78 which was significant well beyond the .01 level. However, nine of the hospitals, or 25%, yielded chi-squares less than 5.99 or the .05 level of significance.

Because the chance of type two errors, failure to reject the null hypothesis when in fact it is false, are decreased by increased sample size, a first hypothesis to explain failures of replication dealt with sample size. The nine hospitals not yielding significant associations between marital status and frequency of early release had an average sample size of 154.0 cases with a standard deviation of 67.78, while the 27 hospitals at which significant associations had been obtained had an average of 247.2 cases with a standard deviation of 102.5. This difference between the size of the samples was significant at the .01 level ($t = 2.98$).

A significant gain from a predictor implies that there is something to predict. The limiting cases are hospitals in which every person achieves an early FSR and hospitals where no one achieves an early FSR. While the latter case has not been obtained empirically, Deiter *et al.* (1964) do in fact report an instance where less than one-half of one per cent of the population would *not* have obtained an early FSR by our present definition. In this case the predictor variables as used here would be valueless. Another example in which the present use of predictor variables would have been of little value is presented by Solomon (1951, table 3, p. 15) in which 90% of 185 committed psychotics had hospital durations of less than six months.

To obtain some empirical notion of the potential interaction of effectiveness of hospitals and strength of predictor variables, Table 4 was devised. The steps by which the table was brought about are too lengthy and too far removed from the major point of this work

TABLE 4. *The association between hospital effectiveness in terms of rate of early FSR and predictive value of different marital statuses for 36 hospitals*

| | Predictive difference marital statuses 1 and 3 | |
|---|---|---|
| | Low=.256 or less | High=.260 and greater |
| Most effective hospitals | 15 | 0 |
| Moderately effective hospitals | 1 | 11 |
| Least effective hospitals | 5 | 4 |

Chi-square, 2 degrees of freedom, $=23.06$; $p<.001$.

to detail and the steps taken will be summarized. To avoid the effect of differing numbers of cases, the difference between marital status 1 (married, notify wife in case of emergency) and marital status 3 (never married) was obtained. The effectiveness of each hospital was ascertained by determining the percentage of early FSR for the patients in marital statuses 1 and 3, and a correction (similar in procedure to the ones in later work to be presented below) was made. To avoid capitalization on chance, a first table dealt with the 12 most effective, the next 12, and the least effective 12 hospitals, i.e. the sample was arbitrarily trisected. The result was a chi-square beyond the .001 level of significance. Next a Moses Test of Extreme Reaction was computed (Siegel, 1956) and found to be significant at the .03 level. Having taken these precautionary steps Table 4 was devised. The point of Table 4 is that the association between the predictor variable and effectiveness was curvilinear.

### *Summary of findings of "marital investigation"*

A strong predictor variable was identified, but a dilemma was also posed. The predictor variable and effectiveness of the hospital were not independent of each other. Either the correction and the measure of effectiveness would be confounded or the difficult assumption that marital status meant different things at different hospitals would have to be made. This difficult choice did not have to be made, because, as will be detailed below, later data indicated that the correction did not alter the ranking of hospitals.

## A STUDY OF EFFECTIVENESS OVER TIME

On methodological grounds, it was necessary to determine the extent to which hospitals were consistent over time in their relative effectiveness. If such test–retest reliability could not be demonstrated, the degree to which the results could be used for making either theoretical or administrative decisions would be reduced. A second important issue involved the not infrequently held belief that routinely compiled records are not as valid as special, *in vivo* personal interviews and follow-ups. Operationally, the purpose of this study was to determine the degree of association between the findings of the PEP study's *in vivo* procedures for patients admitted between September, 1956 through September, 1957, and the findings of the present research from records for men admitted between July 1, 1959 and June 30, 1960.

### *Procedures*

The procedures used by the PEP study were detailed in our summary in Chapter 4. In brief, 1250 patients from 12 hospitals comprised the sample for developing an FSR score. This measure of effectiveness was used both in a "raw" form and in a corrected form after 64 predictor items had been taken into account by covariance.

In the present study, there were 2597 cases collected from the 12 PEP hospitals. The 24 hospitals which remained from the original total of 36 were used to cross-validate the correction variables and avoid capitalization on chance. In addition to marital status, age was used as a predictor variable. The procedure used was identical with the one used in the focal study (see Table 6 and the subsection in Chapter 6 entitled Correction Procedures). For present purposes, we wish to emphasize that data from the 24 "other" hospitals were used to develop a prediction applied to the 12 PEP hospitals.

### *Findings*

For 12 hospitals, uncorrected per cent early FSR yielded an odd-even corrected correlation of .79 for the PEP study sample of 1250 patients,[1] while for the sample of 2597 patients in the present study the corrected odd–even correlation was .89. This difference in reliability was to be expected with the larger sample used in the present procedure compared to the PEP study.

Whereas 61.5% of the PEP sample started an early FSR on or before 274 calendar days after admission, 58.3% of the cases in the present study had started an early FSR by this date.

The correlation between corrected and uncorrected FSR criterion scores was .99 for data collected in the present study. For the PEP study, the corresponding correlation between corrected and uncorrected FSR scores was .91.

The correlation between uncorrected measures of effectiveness (FSR) by the PEP and present studies was .87. The correlation between corrected PEP and present measures of hospital effectiveness was .78. Both correlations were significant past the .001 level with one-tail test. Considering the existence of error of measurement (reflected in odd–even correlations less than unity), the correlation

[1] See table 6, *ibid.*

between uncorrected measures of effectiveness is close to the maximum obtainable correlation. The test–retest measures indicate a high degree of stability in terms of the absolute magnitude of the correlations, significance of the obtained correlations, and the degree to which the correlations approximate the maximum obtainable association.

A matter of interest both statistically and sociologically is the stability over time of the correction factor. On a statistical level, was the raw release rate a function of stability in favorability of sample? On a sociological level, did certain hospitals, for whatever reasons, consistently obtain favorable cases? The answer to these questions is a definite "No." The correlation between the PEP study and the present study's favorability of samples entering hospitals was .10 which was statistically insignificant.

The next question to be answered with these data is whether the two methods at two points in time arrive at similar decisions with regard to the major hypotheses dealing with size, staffing, and effectiveness. Both size and staffing are hospital characteristics which are very stable over time. In a matrix of intercorrelations of size during five successive years,[1] the lowest value found was .98. Similarly, with staffing for five successive years,[2] the lowest correlation was .93, and more than half were .99.

TABLE 5. *Product–moment correlations between size and staffing and PEP and present study raw (uncorrected) and corrected FSR criterion scores**

| | Size (ADPL) | | Staff (FTE/ADPL) | | Size hold staff constant | | Staff hold size constant |
|---|---|---|---|---|---|---|---|
| | *r* | *z* | *r* | *z* | *r* | *z* | *r* |
| PEP study (raw) | −.66 | 2.38 | .51 | 1.69 | −.48 | 1.48 | .07 |
| PEP study (corr.) | −.62 | 2.22 | .43 | 1.38 | −.50 | 1.57 | −.05 |
| present study (raw) | −.64 | 2.27 | .54 | 1.81 | −.42 | 1.28 | .14 |
| present study (corr.) | −.64 | 2.27 | .55 | 1.86 | −.42 | 1.28 | .15 |

*Partials and critical ratios (*z*) computed using correlations to three places.

Correlations between FSR measures of effectiveness and hospital characteristics of size and staffing for 12 hospitals are summarized

[1] See table 2.2, Mimeographed Intramural Report 64–2, *Empirical Dimensions of Hospital Operation: I. Reliability*, prepared by the Psychiatric Evaluation Project, VA Hospital, Washington 7, D.C., July, 1964.

[2] See table 5.1c, *ibid.*

in Table 5. The correlations between uncorrected FSR measures and size are —.66 and —.64 for the PEP and present study's procedures respectively. The correlations between *corrected* FSR measures and size are —.62 and —.64 for the PEP and present study's procedures, respectively. In all cases the correlations are in the predicted direction and significant well past the .02 level with one-tail test. The narrow range of these correlations, between .62 and .66, underlines the similarity of results obtained by the two different procedures at two different periods of time.

The correlations between *uncorrected* FSR scores and staffing per patient were .51 and .54 respectively for the PEP and present study's procedures. The correlations between *corrected* FSR scores and staffing per patient were .43 and .55 respectively for the PEP and present study's procedures. All four of these correlations were in the predicted direction, and three of the four were at the .05 level with one-tail test. The correlation of .43 between staffing and corrected PEP study scores was at the .10 level of significance with one-tail test. Again, the two methods arrive at highly similar statistical decisions.

An important consideration, however, is that the correlation between size and staffing was not random. Rather, size and staffing in the sample of twelve hospitals were inversely associated, the product-moment correlation being —.73. To obtain a clear picture of the association between the effectiveness score and either size or staffing, it was necessary to hold one characteristic constant by means of partial correlation while investigating the other. A sample of 12 cases severely limits this enterprise because of the small number of cases. However, this procedure was undertaken, and the results are presented in Table 5. Holding staffing constant, the correlations between size and effectiveness were significant at the .10 level with one-tail test. On the other hand, the correlations between effectiveness and staffing were random when size was held constant by means of partial correlation.

### *Discussion*

The scores based on procedures using records were highly correlated with the scores obtained by more elaborate *in vivo* procedures. In terms of data on which to base decisions, the two methods arrived at essentially identical results. As such, the procedure to be used in the present study obtained strong empirical validation. Given this validation, a larger number of hospitals than the 12 of the PEP study were investigated and it was possible to explicate the effects of size *or* staffing with the other variable held constant by partial correlation. This work will be reported in the next chapter.

A point which deserves to be emphasized at this time is that having demonstrated the value of a technique for the evaluation of hospital organizations from records, it seems reasonable to hope that the method will be used in studies other than the present one. The technique might conceivably be used in the routine, continuing assessment of hospital effectiveness. Changes such as increased professional staffing, utilization of unit system plans, and the development of special programs might all be measured, with relatively little cost, by the procedures presented in this study.

The use of records has advantages beyond that of lower cost. Once the system has been devised and validated, implementation is a clerical task with a minimum of examiner bias. In an *in vivo* study, the identification of the patient as an object of special study and the additional interviews with professional personnel may well change the very object of study. An *in vivo* study which compares hospitals will usually need to have different research personnel at the different hospitals. There may be a confounding of the particular hospital and the research worker at that hospital. There is evidence (Ullmann, 1961) that such an effect may have occurred in the PEP study. The range of PEP patients found untestable upon admission ranged from 3.8% to 35.2% across the 12 hospital-psychologists involved. It was impossible to say whether the difference in rate of untestability (which yielded a chi-square of 74.31 where, for 11 degrees of freedom, a chi-square of 31.26 is significant at the .001 level) was due to the type of patients admitted to each hospital or the psychologist at that hospital.

The magnitude of the .87 correlation between uncorrected percentage of FSR at the 12 PEP hospitals as measured by the PEP study and the present study, appears in retrospect as remarkably high. The matter of the less than perfect odd–even reliability of the two measures has already been mentioned. In our summary of the PEP study, we noted that one of the hospitals underwent structural changes during the intake period of the PEP study and we should note that a different hospital underwent changes in size and staffing during part of the present study. Finally, of greatest importance, is the fact that the two studies used somewhat different procedures. These differences were in scoring procedures, sampling, and corrections for potential differences in samples admitted to different hospitals.

In the present study from records, if a man died after continuous hospitalization of 275 or more days, he was considered a late FSR because he had failed to establish an early FSR and had been unequivocally classified prior to his death. Again, if he left the hospital on day 100 and remained in the community steadily until his death on day 200, he had unequivocally established an early FSR and was kept in the sample. Only if he was transferred or died before clearly establishing either an early or late FSR was the patient removed from the sample. In the PEP study, however, the man was excluded from the sample if he died at any time in four years or was transferred directly from his admitting hospital any time during the four years. Some of the PEP study patients would have established unequivocal early FSRs, others unequivocal late FSRs, while others would have been indeterminate. Another difference in procedure was that in the PEP study, if the man left the hospital other than by direct transfer and entered another hospital, his remaining off the census was sufficient to obtain an early FSR. That is, if a man left on day 270 and entered a different hospital on day 300, the case was equivocal and dropped in the present work while in the PEP study this outcome would have been considered an early FSR.

While the PEP study used men with any functional psychosis the present study was limited to schizophrenic reaction. In the PEP study, men were included only if they had been in the community at least 90 of the preceding 180 days. The present study did not have this restriction and used all men who were newly admitted, under 60 years of age, and diagnosed as schizophrenic. In contrast to the PEP study, in the present work to rule out administrative admissions, at least seven calendar days had to intervene between admission and start of the first significant release.

Another major difference in the sampling was that in the present study all admissions during a total year were used. In the PEP study, as previously noted, when the quota of patients had been achieved, intake ceased. At some hospitals this meant an intake procedure covering seven months, at other hospitals a procedure covering 12 months. This is relevant because in the present study there is evidence that admissions to psychiatric hospitals are not uniform over the calendar year. Across the 8060 cases at the 36 hospitals evaluated by the present procedure, the six-month period from November through April saw fewer admissions ($t = 4.59$; $p = .001$). However, a higher percentage of the admissions during these months obtained an early FSR ($t = 6.54$; $p < .001$). There are many difficulties with the interpretation of these data, but the point is the greater empirical appropriateness, logic, and generalizability followed in the sampling of the present work. In the PEP study hospitals which rapidly filled their quotas drew more heavily on the November through April months, those of higher FSR rate, a matter which introduced an unmeasured source of error.

The problem of correction for possible variations among samples entering different hospitals was approached in dissimilar ways by the two studies. As noted in our earlier quotation from Cohen (1964), the PEP study used an analysis of variance with 64 covariates. It is possible to wonder how these 64 items were selected so that capitalization on chance was avoided, the degree to which this many items were independent and avoided repeated measure of the same variance, and the effects of unreliability of 64 variables in a covariance design. In short, the PEP study made use of an elaborate procedure which involved complex statistical assumptions. It is possible to wonder whether such procedures were theoretically justified, empirically necessary, and might not have introduced error into the statistical decision they were designed to facilitate. In contrast, the present study used a simpler procedure (both in number of variables and method of application) and developed a correction score from 24 hospitals independent of the 12 investigated in this preliminary research. Particularly in a cross-validated design, it is crucial to note that the correlation between hospitals ordered with and without correction was .99.

### *Summary of a study of effectiveness over time*

Two procedures were used to study the same 12 hospitals at different periods of time. The results indicate that the use of records provided results which were essentially identical with those obtained from an *in vivo* study both in the absolute correlation coefficient and in the statistical decisions relevant to the association of size and staffing with effectiveness. These findings validate the procedures for use with an enlarged sample of hospitals.

## CHAPTER 6

# *The Focal Study of Size and Staffing*

IN THIS chapter we will directly test the association of size and staffing of psychiatric hospitals with the effectiveness of these hospitals. As was noted in the two previous chapters, size and staffing are likely to be significantly correlated with each other. It is therefore necessary to hold one variable constant by means of partial correlation when determining the relationship of the other to criterion measures of effectiveness. Such a procedure requires a larger number of cases than the 12 used in the PEP study. If a more complete analysis is not presented we cannot say whether the significant correlation between staffing and FSR is due to the presumptive value of staffing or the favorable staffing pattern at small hospitals. An example of how some third variable may underlie and offer an alternative explanation to a presumed relationship is an article by Cohen and Struening (1964) which asserts that authoritarian-restrictive attitudes on the part of the staff "caused" low effectiveness when the results could have been as easily, if not more easily, explained on the basis of the size of the hospitals (Ullmann, 1965).

## PROCEDURES

### *Selection of hospitals*

At the time of the present study, there were 40 VA hospitals with major psychiatric missions. Because we were interested in determining the effects of size and staffing patterns with measures of the effectiveness of the treatment of psychiatric patients, certain hospitals were ruled out of the focal analysis because their inclusion would have introduced difficulties in the assessment of these variables.

The primary variable which led to the exclusion of certain hospitals was a major general medical and surgical treatment program. In our summary of the PEP study in Chapter 4 we cited Davis (1964) to the effect that factor analyses of psychiatric hospitals revealed general medical and surgical treatment to be the second factor, after size, accounting for differences among hospital characteristics. In preliminary studies for the present work, it was found that the greater the proportion of beds devoted to nonpsychiatric cases, the greater was the expense per patient per day. Because the length of hospital stay of general medical patients is usually considerably shorter than the stay of psychiatric patients, using 40 VA hospitals with major psychiatric missions, the following .80 correlations were found: between proportion of general medical patients and expense, between proportion of general medical patients and turnover, and between turnover and expense. The situation called for, at minimum, the use of partial correlation. However, this was a situation in which statistical control would be only as adequate as the data available, and data indicating how much money was actually spent on psychiatric patients and how much was actually spent on general medical patients were not available. That is, a breakdown of expenditure within hospitals for types of patients, as distinct from number and type of employees, was not available. A second factor was that from my personal observations at a hospital in which general medical involvement increased sharply in what had previously been a hospital devoted exclusively to psychiatric treatment, qualitative as well as quantitative considerations may be involved. The orientation and professional bases for decision-making of psychiatrists differ from those of other medical specialists. The non-psychiatrist has a patient who is in a life-and-death emergency situation where the psychiatric patient will survive another day, another week, another month, another year. General medical treatment had a higher priority on available funds than psychiatric treatment such that as the hospital's staff to patient ratio increased, psychiatric staffing, particularly for continued treatment patients, decreased sharply. Staffing of some psychiatric wards became so thin as to reach the point of literal danger.

It is my opinion that the struggle for funds is curvilinear with relation to the proportion of either general medical or psychiatric patients. If the overwhelming proportion of patients, and therefore physicians, are psychiatric, they can hold their own and be, essentially, in control. If the overwhelming proportion of patients are in the general medical group, i.e. the hospital is a "general medical" rather than "psychiatric" hospital, psychiatry then represents such a small part of the available funds that the psychiatric service can approach the staffing pattern of the other medical specialties without a major budgetary struggle. A rate of expenditure similar to other medical specialties is, for psychiatric endeavors, unusually high and favorable. The development of small psychiatric wards within general hospitals are examples of this. It is only when the proportion of either of the two types of medical missions becomes sizable that a struggle is likely to ensue. Based on both theoretical grounds and an inspection of the hospitals available for study, a minimum ratio of at least seven-eighths (87.5%) of the average daily patient load (ADPL) being psychiatric was set. This cut-off permitted physicians whose major interest was the care and treatment of psychiatric patients to be in an overwhelming majority at the hospitals.

Given this rule, four hospitals with major nonpsychiatric missions were excluded from all data collection and analyses. This left the 36 hospitals which were evaluated by the data collection procedures of the present work. However, as noted in Chapter 4, three of the original 12 PEP hospitals had major nonpsychiatric missions and a fourth underwent changes in size, patient characteristics, and staffing pattern immediately after the intake period of the present study. From the beginning of the study, these hospitals were excluded from plans for the focal study to be presented in this and the following chapter. However, because these hospitals were among the twelve studied by PEP, all the data of the present work were collected from these hospitals and used in the second preliminary study reported in Chapter 5.

Two hospitals which were to have been in the focal sample were excluded when less than 100 clear early or late FSR designations were obtained at each. Because the FSR score for each hospital is a percentage, it was arbitrarily decided that there should be at least 100 cases in the denominator for each hospital.

In short, situations which might have led to confounding the measures were dealt with at a first level by means of sample selection. What remained were the 30 psychiatric hospitals of the focal sample: all the VA psychiatric hospitals except those which (a) had a major nonpsychiatric mission; (b) had undergone major structural (size) changes during the study period; or (c) had fewer than a total of 100 patients establishing unequivocal FSR designations.

### *Sample of patients*

For the 30 hospitals in this sample there were 7212 male schizophrenics under age 60 who unequivocally established an early or late FSR. The number of cases at each hospital ranged from 113 to 538 with an average of 240. In terms of type of schizophrenic reaction, 37.4% were paranoid, 7.4% catatonic, 3.9% hebephrenic, 1.9% simple, 3.2% schizo-affective, 1.2% residual, and the remainder, 45.0% undifferentiated. Description of the sample in terms of marital status and age may be found in Table 6 and is an integral part of the correction procedure to be discussed in the immediately succeeding paragraphs.

### *Correction procedures*

The purpose of a correction procedure was discussed in connection with the first preliminary study presented in Chapter 5. As in that work, three categories of marital status were used. In the first category, comprising 29.6% of the 7212 patients, were the men who were married and who listed their wives as the people to notify in case of emergency. Of this group, 74.1% established an early FSR. The second category was composed of men who had married at some time in their lives but who did not list a wife as the person to notify in case of emergency. This group, which included primarily the divorced and widowed, comprised 21.3% of the patient sample, and 62.8% of these cases established an early FSR. The third category was composed of the men who had never married. This category accounted for 49.1% of the sample, and within it 48.4% established an early FSR. The chi-square, with two degrees of freedom, was 377.98 indicating a highly significant association between marital status and early FSR. Age was investigated to determine whether it would significantly *add* to the prediction obtained from marital status alone. The sample was divided into three age groups: from 17 to 30, from 31 to 45, and from 46 to 59 years of age.[1] As presented in Table 6, each of the three marital statuses was subdivided into the three age

[1] To determine whether a finer discrimination would be worthwhile, each age category was further subdivided. There were not enough extremely young or extremely old patients to warrant further computation, and there was no significant predictive difference between the 31–37- and the 38–45-year-old age groups.

levels. Within all three marital categories, younger age was associated with more favorable prognosis to an extent well past the .001 level of significance.

TABLE 6. *The association between early FSR and categorization by marital status and age for 7212 schizophrenic admissions*

MARRIED, NOTIFY WIFE

| | Early FSR | Late FSR | Sum | % early FSR |
|---|---|---|---|---|
| Age 17–30 | 266 | 67 | 333 | 79.9 |
| Age 31–45 | 1163 | 397 | 1560 | 74.6 |
| Age 46–59 | 155 | 89 | 244 | 63.5 |
| Sum | 1584 | 553 | 2137 | |

Chi-square, 2*df*, = 20.16; $p < .001$.

MARRIED, NOTIFY SOMEONE OTHER THAN WIFE

| | Early FSR | Late FSR | Sum | % early FSR |
|---|---|---|---|---|
| Age 17–30 | 147 | 63 | 210 | 70.0 |
| Age 31–45 | 710 | 400 | 1110 | 64.0 |
| Age 46–59 | 106 | 108 | 214 | 49.5 |
| Sum | 963 | 571 | 1534 | |

Chi-square, 2*df*, = 21.57; $p < .001$.

NEVER MARRIED

| | Early FSR | Late FSR | Sum | % early FSR |
|---|---|---|---|---|
| Age 17–30 | 684 | 577 | 1261 | 54.2 |
| Age 31–45 | 898 | 1050 | 1948 | 46.1 |
| Age 46–59 | 132 | 200 | 332 | 39.8 |
| Sum | 1714 | 1827 | 3541 | |

Chi-square, 2*df*, = 30.96; $p < .001$.

As in previous work, a first FSR criterion score was simply the percentage of cases at each hospital achieving an early FSR. The score, which may be called raw FSR, varied for the 30 hospitals from 41.4% achieving an early FSR to 74.7% with an average of 57.9%.

For purposes of correcting for potential sampling differences, the following technique, which was also used in the first preliminary study reported in Chapter 5 was devised. The number of cases at each hospital falling into each age–marital status category was multiplied by the proportion of men in that category achieving an early FSR. The products for each of the nine categories were summed. This sum was divided by the number of cases at each hospital and became the base rate or expected percentage of early FSR for that hospital. The expected percentage of early FSR was subtracted from the percentage of early FSR actually obtained at each hospital, and after a constant had been added to eliminate negative numbers, the resulting figure was the corrected FSR score. This score ranged from hospitals obtaining 16% fewer to hospitals obtaining 16% more FSR than would have been expected on the basis of the proportion of men in each age–marital status admitted to each hospital.

The correlation between the raw and corrected FSR scores at the 30 hospitals was .99. This indicated that the two measures were virtually identical and that the correction procedure altered the scores of relative effectiveness of the hospitals to a negligible extent. From this finding, it seemed unlikely that additional corrections for potential differences among samples would lead to major changes in the correlations between FSR criteria and measures of size or staffing.

Because they were so similar, only one FSR measure would be useful and not redundant. Therefore, in further work, unless otherwise noted, only the FSR measure corrected for age and marital status will be used. The selection of the corrected FSR score was decided upon as follows: those readers who were statistically sophisticated would recognize the essential identity of the two measures and consider which of the two was chosen a matter of indifference. On the other hand, those readers who were less familiar with statistical procedures might still wonder about the matter of correction, and for their benefit, the corrected measure was selected.

### *Additional remarks on FSR measurement characteristics*

With a sample of 30 hospitals, the odd–even correlation for raw FSR scores was .92 (after use of Spearman–Brown formula). Despite the increased number of cases, this was a slight increase over the correlation reported for the 12 PEP hospitals. It is not unlikely that this increase was a result of the more careful selection of hospitals as well as the larger minimum number of cases at each hospital.

As previously noted, an early FSR was a release lasting at least 90 days which started on or by the 274th calendar day after admission. Because FSR is a cumulative measure, i.e. a person who establishes an FSR by a given date retains that accomplishment thereafter, it is not surprising hospital effectiveness as measured by percentages of early FSR by 90 days or 180 days after admission should be very highly correlated with percentage of early FSR by 274 calendar days after admission. It was found that the correlation for 30 hospitals between FSR percentage by 90 days after admission and 274 days after admission was .92. The correlation between FSR percentage by 180 days and by 274 days after admission was .97.

A more sophisticated analysis, however, deals with the question of the correlation of percentage of FSR *of those cases remaining* (not having established an early FSR) in each time period. To do this, those patients who had achieved an early FSR during the first three months were removed from both the numerator and the denominator. This investigation also gives some greater detail as to when, in terms of admission, early FSRs started. Of the total of 7212 cases in the 30 hospital sample, 414 (or 5.74%) cases started their early FSRs on or before the 30th day after admission; 773 cases (or 10.72% of the total sample) started their early FSR between the 31st and 60th day after admission; and 747 cases (or 10.36% of the total sample) started their early FSR between the 61st and 90th day after admission. In sum, 1934 out of 7212 patients, or 26.82% of the sample, started their early FSRs within 90 days after admission. Between the 91st and 180th day after admission, 1521 patients started their early FSR. This represents 21.09% of the total sample of 7212 cases; however, when the 1934 cases who had started an early FSR by the 90th day after admission were removed from the sample, 5278 cases remained as of the 91st day after admission. *Of the cases remaining* 28.82% started an early FSR between the 91st and 180th day after admission. Between the 181st and 274th day after admission 806 cases started their early FSRs. This is 11.18% of the total sample of 7212 cases, but it is 21.45% of the 3757 cases remaining on the 181st day after admission, i.e. who had not started an early FSR previously. It is interesting to note that *when the total sample is taken into account, the percentage of patients establishing an early FSR is negatively accelerated mainly because the number of patients remaining who can, by chance, establish an early FSR is sharply reduced.*

Of prime interest is the correlation for the 30 hospitals between percentages of early FSR established during successive three month periods based on those cases remaining. The correlation for 30 hospitals between the percentage of patients establishing an early FSR during the first 90 days after admission ($N = 7212$) and the percentage of those patients *remaining* on the 91st day ($N = 5278$) who established an FSR between the 91st and 180th day was .76. The correlation for 30 hospitals between the percentage of patients remaining on the 91st day who established an early FSR between the 91st and 180th day after admission, and the percentage of the patients ($N = 3757$) remaining on the 181st day after admission who established an early FSR between the 181st and 274th day after admission was .56. Finally, the correlation for 30 hospitals between percentages of patients establishing an early FSR by the 90th day, and the percentage (of those remaining on the 181st day after admission) of patients who established an FSR between the 181st and 274th day after admission was .57. All three of these correlations are significant at or beyond the .001 level. These correlations indicate that at least for three-fourths of a year, *good hospitals were good.* There is a stability of the FSR effectiveness measure at different time periods. That such stability was obtained was all the more impressive for two reasons.

The first reason was that each time those cases who had established an early FSR were removed, the number of cases, and hence the consistency of the measure, was reduced. The number of cases remaining on which to establish an early FSR percentage during the period from the 181st through the 274th day after admission was only slightly more than half (52%) of the number of cases available for the denominator for percentage of early FSR by the 90th day. Another way of saying this is that for the final period, the denominator of number of cases remaining was less than 100 for 11 of the 30 hospitals, and in one instance was as low as 44 cases.

The second reason was, perhaps, conceptually more important. The hospital with a low percentage of early FSR cases in the first period presumably had more "good bets" available during the next period than did the hospital in which such men had already established an early FSR. Given this circumstance, negative rather than positive correlations would be expected. The better hospitals maintained higher percentages of early FSRs in successive periods, even though this was done with proportionately smaller and presumably more difficult segments of the total sample.

### *Additional measures of effectiveness*

The measure of FSR deals with the percentage of male schizophrenic patients under 60 who after starting a new admission achieved a significant release within a limited period of time. It is a measure of the percentage of admitted patients who are benefited relatively rapidly. But efforts continue and a second general area of effectiveness is the degree to which hospitals avoid a build-up of long-term patients. This general area will be called *turnover* and empirical evidence why it is so labeled will be forthcoming. There are conceivably three points at which turnover may be measured: first at intake, in which high turnover is reflected by a high intake of patients per size (number of beds); second, at exit, in which the number of terminated cases per unit size is the measure; and finally, the number of cases who remain continuously in the hospital. This third and last measure recalls Jones and Sidebotham's comment that their large hospital, Northtown, was essentially two hospitals, one large and static, the other small and with rapid turnover. Low turnover and, particularly, a high percentage of men with long, continuous hospitalizations, may serve to tap the extent to which there is present this second, static population.

Given this background a first additional criterion measure of effectiveness was a measure of *intake per unit size* (intake/size). This measure was the total number of schizophrenic cases in this study from each hospital who established an early *or* late FSR divided by the size of the patient population at that hospital. Intake/size has the advantages of (a) being restricted to a single diagnostic group, schizophrenic reaction; (b) being protected against any patient being counted more than once; and (c) eliminating errors due to death or transfer to another hospital prior to the clear designation of an early or late FSR. That is, this criterion, intake/size, was free of the most common criticisms of turnover figures. For the 30 hospitals, the range was from 8.0% to 38.2% with an average of 17.8%.

A different criterion measure came from the *VA Field Station Summaries* and was a more typical measure of *turnover*. In these routinely compiled reports, the number of psychiatric cases terminated in a given period are divided by the size of the patient population. Whereas the previous criterion, intake/size, dealt with admissions and was restricted to schizophrenic reactions, the present turnover measure dealt with termination (discharge, death, and transfer) for all diagnostic categories. Turnover is reported quarterly. The four quarters of each of the two years (fiscal years 1960 and 1961) of this study were separately summed. The correlation between turnover in the successive years was .95 for the sample of 30 hospitals, indicating a high degree of stability over time. For criterion purposes, turnover in the two successive years was averaged. The range of this *%-turnover* figure was from 8.80% per annum to 37.85% per annum with an average of 17.12%.

A final criterion measure was percentage of patients with relatively *long hospital residence.* This figure was obtained from the *VA Field Station Summaries* where once a year information was collected on a 20% sample of all patients in VA hospitals. The measure chosen for this study was the percentage of patients in hospitals who had been in residence two or more years (% 2+ years). The per cent whose residence had been two or more years at each hospital was correlated for successive years. This correlation was .90, indicating stability over time. To arrive at the criterion measure used in the present research, the figures for the two successive years were averaged. For the 30 hospitals in the sample, the range of percentage of patients with two or more years residence was from 50.0% to 82.0% with an average of 71.6%.

### *Hospital size and staffing*

The purpose of this research was to determine the association between size, staffing, and hospital effectiveness. *Hospital size* was determined from the *VA Field Station Summaries* report of ADPL, Average Daily Patient Load, during the two fiscal years of this study. The correlation between ADPL for one year with ADPL during the succeeding year was .999. That is, size was a highly stable characteristic during the period of study. The size figures (ADPL) for the two years were averaged and became the measure of size used in the present study. The range of size (ADPL) for the 30 hospitals was from 604 to 2390 patients, with an average of 1453.

To obtain an overall figure regarding *staffing*, data in the *VA Field Station Summaries* were again used. Here, the number of Full Time Equivalents (FTE), a method for correcting for number of part-time workers, is reported each month. Figures were obtained for three months: June, 1959, June, 1960, and June, 1961, marking the beginning, middle, and end of the study period. Each hospital's number of FTEs was divided by the size of the hospital. The inter-correlations of these three figures were .93, .96, and .96 indicating a high degree of stability over time. The average of the three figures (FTE/ADPL) became the measure of staffing used in the present study. At the 30 hospitals the number of employees per patient ranged from .594 to 1.145 with an average of .705.

### *Hospital psychiatric involvement*

A final hospital characteristic which was taken into account was the degree of psychiatric involvement. In the present study, hospitals with a high nonpsychiatric mission, i.e. tuberculosis, general medicine, neurology/geriatrics, were eliminated. The measure used was the number of psychiatric cases divided by the total average daily patient load. This figure was derived for each of the 30 hospitals from three successive reports, i.e. June, 1959, June, 1960, and June, 1961, the beginning, middle, and end of the study period. The intercorrelations between the figures were .98, .94, and .97. In short, this characteristic, even when an attenuated sample had been selected, was stable over time. The three figures were averaged to provide the measure called *%-psychiatric* in the present research. The range was from 87% of the inpatient population designated as psychiatric to 100% with an average of 96.5%.

## RESULTS

Table 7 presents the basic findings of this study. The first four columns of Table 7 deal with the measures of effectiveness, the next two columns deal with size as measured by average daily patient load, ADPL, and staffing as measured by number of full time employees per patient, FTE/ADPL. The final two columns deal with per cent psychiatric involvement and the correlation between staffing ratio (FTE/size) and the other variables in the matrix with per cent psychiatric involvement held constant by means of partial correlation.

TABLE 7. *Intercorrelation of four measures of hospital effectiveness, size and staffing for 30 psychiatric hospitals*

| | 1 | 2 | 3 | 4 | 5 | 6 | 7 | 8* |
|---|---|---|---|---|---|---|---|---|
| 1. FSR | .. | .55 | .65 | −.49 | −.37 | .15 | .06 | .20 |
| 2. Intake/size | | .. | .80 | −.84 | −.46 | .66 | .04 | .77 |
| 3. %-turnover | | | .. | −.88 | −.39 | .48 | .07 | .57 |
| 4. % 2+ years' stay | | | | .. | .51 | −.73 | .12 | −.74 |
| 5. Size | | | | | .. | −.44 | −.06 | −.53 |
| 6. FTE/size (staffing) | | | | | | .. | −.46 | .. |
| 7. %-psychiatric | | | | | | | .. | .. |

*Column 8 deals with FTE/size to variables 1–6 with variable number 7, %-psychiatric, held constant by partial correlation.

### *Effect of varying per cent psychiatric*

To avoid confounding results dealing with psychiatric patients when the hospital had a major nonpsychiatric mission, hospitals had been selected which had a high percentage of psychiatric patients composing the average daily patient load. Even with such attenuation, the variations in percentage of psychiatric patients (%-psychiatric) were highly stable over time. From column 7 of Table 7, it may be noted that the %-psychiatric variable was significantly associated only with the staffing per patient measure. As %-psychiatric patients increased, the staffing ratio decreased. The final column of Table 7 presents partial correlations to hold constant the effect of %-psychiatric (McNemar, 1962, p. 166). As may be noted, the effect was to increase the correlations between staffing per patient and measures of effectiveness, but in no case did a previously insignificant correlation become statistically significant.

### *The correlation between size and staffing*

As reported in Table 7, the correlation between size and staffing was statistically significant, —.44. As hospitals became smaller, in the present sample, they tended to have more staff per patient. Because this was so, there was empirical evidence for the need to use partial correlation to hold one characteristic, size or staffing, constant while determining the relationship of the other to measures of effectiveness.

### *Intercorrelation among measures of turnover*

There were three measures of turnover. The first was the %-turnover figure obtained directly from the *VA Field Station Summaries*. The second measure was the per cent of patients in the hospital whose stay was two or more years (% 2+ years' stay). The third measure was the number of cases establishing an FSR (early or late) at each hospital divided by the size of that hospital (intake/size). Where %-turnover was a measure at exit, % 2+ years' stay was a measure of static population, and intake/size was a measure at admission. From Table 7 it may be noted that there was empirical evidence that these three criteria were measuring essentially the same construct. The correlation between intake/size and %-turnover was .80. The correlation between intake/size and % 2+ years' stay was —.84 (i.e. high intake/size associated with low % 2+ years' stay), and the correlation between %-turnover and % 2+ years' stay was —.88.

### *Relationship between FSR and three turnover measures*

It is logical that measures of effectiveness, in general, be significantly associated. In particular, it may be hypothesized that the more early releases there are, the greater will be the space available for intake of new patients, the lower will be the percentage of inpatients with long stay, and the higher will be turnover as measured by terminated cases. From Table 7 it may be noted that this was in fact the case. All the correlations among criteria were in the predicted direction and significant beyond the .01 level. However, while the three measures of the turnover construct were significantly associated with the early release measure, it was possible to determine that these scores were measuring something different from and in addition to early release. Specifically, when FSR was held constant by means of partial correlation, the correlation between %-turnover and % 2+ years' stay decreased minimally from —.88 to —.84; the correlation between intake/size and % 2+ years' stay decreased from —.84 to

—.78; and the correlation between %-turnover and intake/size decreased from .80 to .70. This last correlation, the lowest of the triad, yielded a critical ratio of 4.42, significant well beyond the .001 level, and therefore, the three measures of turnover were very significantly intercorrelated even when FSR was held constant.

### *The relationship between favorable outcome and size and staffing*

With 30 cases, a correlation of .32 or greater is needed to reject the null hypothesis at the .05 level with one-tail test ($z = 1.65$). From Table 7, it may be noted that the correlation between size (ADPL) and FSR was —.37, which was in the predicted direction and statistically significant. That is, to a statistically significant extent, small hospital size was associated with a high percentage of early releases. The correlation between staffing ratio (FTE/ADPL) and FSR was in the predicted (positive) direction but was not statistically significant. Both size and staffing were significantly correlated in the predicted direction with all three criterion measures of turnover.

### *The effect of size or staffing with the other characteristic held constant*

A major strength of the present undertaking was a number of hospitals large enough to permit the use of partial correlation and hence a test of the effect of one characteristic, either size *or* staffing, with the other held constant. Table 8 presents this material.

TABLE 8. *Partial correlations for 30 psychiatric hospitals relating four measures of hospital effectiveness to size* or *staffing*

| | A: size, holding staffing constant | B: staffing, holding size constant |
|---|---|---|
| FSR | −.34* | −.02 |
| Intake/size | −.24 | .57† |
| %-turnover | −.23 | .37* |
| % 2+ years' stay | .30 | −.65† |

* = .05 level, one tail.
† = .001 level.

The data reported in Table 8 indicate that even when staffing was held constant, small size was significantly associated with high early release rate (FSR). There was also a trend, bordering on significance, for small size to be associated with the three measures of turnover after staffing had been held constant. On the other hand, while staffing was randomly associated with early release when size was held constant, high staffing was significantly associated with all three measures of turnover after size had been held constant by means of partial correlation. *The results indicate the demonstrable value of both size and staffing, and, perhaps more importantly, do so in such a manner as to specify the particular beneficial effect each has on different measures of hospital effectiveness.*

## ADDITIONAL COMPUTATIONS

### *Status on discharge*

A number of further analyses were undertaken to deal with questions raised by the preceding information. The first question dealt with the possibility that small hospitals achieved their superior early FSR rates by discharging men in less satisfactory symptomatic condition than large hospitals. While our review of the literature of psychiatric condition at discharge (Jones and Sidebotham, 1962; Odegard, 1961) and the criterion of remaining in the community at least 90 consecutive days would argue against such a concept, an additional bit of information was available. The status on which each man started his FSR had been noted and it was possible to categorize early FSRs as starting on a status *with medical approval* (maximum hospital benefit, MHB; trial visit, TV; or leave of absence, LOA) *or without medical approval* (absence without leave, AWOL; against medical advice, AMA). The hospitals were divided into the 12 with a relatively smaller number of patients (ADPL up to 1201) and the 18 with a relatively large number of patients (ADPL 1316 or more). The cutting point was determined on both an absolute numerical basis and by the fact that a difference of over 100 resident patients separated the largest small hospital from the smallest large hospital. Given the views of the World Health Organization, the Joint Commission on Mental Illness and Health, and the other authorities cited in the introductory material, 1200 patients seemed the maximum justifiable upper limit for a "small" hospital. It was found that the 12 small hospitals not only had a higher percentage of early FSRs, but also a lower percentage of cases starting their early FSRs in one of the "without medical approval" categories. For the "small" hospitals, 14.98% of the early FSRs started without medical approval, while for the "large" hospitals 21.21% of the early FSRs started without medical approval. Given the large number of cases involved, this difference was statistically significant well past the .001 level, the chi-square with one degree of freedom being 25.30.

### *A cohort analysis*

An analysis dealt with the questions of (a) how much smaller hospital size *added* to the prediction obtained from knowledge of age and marital status and (b) whether smaller hospital size was of particular value with particular patients. Table 9 presents this analysis. *For all nine age and marital status categories, smaller hospitals had a higher early FSR rate than larger hospitals.* Smaller hospital size was particularly important with the patient group with the poorest likelihood of early release, the men who had never married.

This mode of analysis will be repeated in Table 16 which makes use of analyses of hospital characteristics additional to those of size. In an analysis such as that presented in Table 9, rather than "correcting," the hypothesis is tested with nine different samples, the nine different age-marital status categories. Age and marital status were held constant by the homogeniety of each group, and the samples were homogeneous in terms of the administrative requirements of admission to a VA hospital and the diagnostic restriction of schizophrenic reaction.

### *Age of hospitals*

It is possible to wonder, particularly with the measure of the percentage of men with two or more years continuous hospitalization, whether the age of the hospital was a significant variable. For example, it might be reasoned that if only a relatively small percentage of men do become prolonged treatment cases, it takes time for a hospital to accumulate a large proportion of chronic cases. If this were so, it would be predicted that there would be a positive correlation between the age of the hospital and the percentage of men with

TABLE 9. *Early release rates (FSR) for schizophrenic admissions at large and small hospitals stratified by age and marital status*

| | Small hospitals | | Large hospitals | | Difference | |
|---|---|---|---|---|---|---|
| | No. cases | % early FSR | No. cases | % early FSR | % early FSR | $X^2$ |
| MARRIED, NOTIFY WIFE | | | | | | |
| Age 17–30 | 122 | 85.25 | 211 | 76.78 | 8.47 | 2.94 |
| Age 31–45 | 569 | 79.96 | 991 | 71.44 | 8.52 | 13.84 |
| Age 46–59 | 91 | 67.03 | 153 | 61.44 | 5.59 | 0.55 |
| MARRIED, NOTIFY OTHER THAN WIFE | | | | | | |
| Age 17–30 | 54 | 75.93 | 156 | 67.95 | 7.98 | 0.87 |
| Age 31–45 | 398 | 66.83 | 712 | 62.36 | 4.47 | 2.03 |
| Age 46–59 | 67 | 50.75 | 147 | 48.98 | 1.77 | 0.09 |
| NEVER MARRIED | | | | | | |
| Age 17–30 | 452 | 59.07 | 809 | 51.55 | 7.52 | 6.31 |
| Age 31–45 | 675 | 53.48 | 1273 | 42.18 | 11.30 | 22.21 |
| Age 46–59 | 108 | 55.56 | 224 | 32.14 | 23.42 | 15.71 |

two or more years' stay. On the other hand, one might reason that when a new hospital within a system is activated, to increase rapidly the resident population, other hospitals in that system will transfer to it some of their patients. It takes little experience in the system to predict that hospitals with the option of sending away some of their patients are not likely to choose their most favorable cases. Given this line of reasoning, it would be predicted that age of hospital would be negatively correlated with the percentage of men with two or more years' stay. In either case, it is possible to expect a significant association between age of the hospital and turnover as measured by percentage of men with two or more years' stay.

All the hospitals in the sample were at least six years old in 1959 at the start of the study. The oldest were 38 years in terms of their operation as psychiatric hospitals by a federal veterans agency. It should be noted that the Veterans Administration as currently constituted did not come into being until 1932, but it should also be noted that some of the structures had been used for various purposes from 1890 onwards. In the present study, the basic data were taken from Hamilton (1944, pp. 163–4), with supplementation for hospitals established after his survey. A final caution is that historically the newer hospitals have tended to be smaller and more highly staffed. It was necessary, therefore, to determine the association between age and hospital characteristics such as size and staffing lest a presumptively significant correlation between age and a criterion measure would in fact be a function of staffing or size.

For the 30 hospitals, the correlation between hospital age and percentage of men with two or more years' stay was statistically significant, .40. However, the correlation between hospital age and staffing was —.47, indicating that indeed the newer hospitals were more highly staffed. As noted in Table 7, the correlation between staffing and percentage of men with two or more years' stay was —.73. *When staffing was held constant by means of partial correlation, the correlation between age and percentage of men with two or more years' stay decreased to statistical insignificance, .10.* When both size and staffing were held constant by means of double-partial correlation (McNemar, 1962, pp. 164–7) the correlation between hospital age and percentage of men with two or more years' hospitalization decreased further to .07.

In similar fashion, the association between age and FSR was investigated. The correlation between age of hospital and FSR was

−.22, which was not statistically significant. The correlation between age and size was .28, which while not statistically significant, did indicate some moderate trend over time for hospitals to become smaller. When staffing was held constant by partial correlation, the correlation between age and FSR dropped to −.17. When both size and staffing were held constant by means of double-partial correlation, the correlation between age of hospital and percentage of early FSR decreased further to −.15. In short, the age of the hospital, other than as it was associated with size and staffing, was not significantly correlated with the criterion measures.

### *Diagnostic practices*

Given the unreliability of psychiatric diagnosis, it is possible to wonder if differential diagnostic practices may not have influenced the number of schizophrenics taken into the sample at each hospital. This would directly affect the turnover measure of intake per size. While the strong intercorrelation between the three measures of turnover (at intake, exit, and continuing resident population) would argue against this concept, the possibility existed. Further, it might be argued that higher staff could lead to more careful diagnostic practices and hence some significant association between staffing and diagnostic practices. Another hypothesis was that the more isolated the hospital was, the more difficult would be its task because urban hospitals would obtain a greater proportion of patients such as neurotics, while rural hospitals would obtain cases for whom the expectation of a relatively long hospitalization made the journey worthwhile.

The procedure for collecting data was as follows: lists of the admission diagnosis for all psychiatric patients during a full year were available. The two major categories of functional psychiatric disorders were schizophrenia and neurosis. A tabulation was made of each time one or the other of these diagnostic categories was assigned upon admission. Unlike other work in the present study, in this instance a man could enter the sample more than once, e.g. due to readmission. This was done because the focus of interest was the relative frequency with which the two diagnostic labels were used.

For the 30 hospitals there was a total of 9303 calls of schizophrenia on admission and a total of 3195 calls of neurosis. The former figure provides some indication of the number of readmissions, transfers, changed diagnoses, etc., which were taken into account by the present procedures for determining FSR. That is, there eventually were 7212 unequivocal FSR designations from a pool of 9303 "schizophrenic" admissions. A final preliminary note is that as the number of schizophrenic calls at a hospital increased, so did the number of neurotic calls. To rule out sheer size of hospital as something which increased the number of both types of diagnoses at larger hospitals, the number of schizophrenic diagnoses and the number of neurotic diagnoses made at each hospital were divided by the average daily patient load (size) of the hospital. When this had been done, the correlation between the number of schizophrenic diagnoses and number of neurotic diagnoses was positive and highly significant, .75. This correlation indicates that a hospital with a high intake per size for schizophrenic diagnoses is also very likely to have a high intake per size for neurotic diagnoses.

Size, and particularly staffing, are associated with the intake per size figure. To evaluate differential diagnostic practices without the influence of size of intake *per se*, the measure investigated took the form of a proportion. The method used was to obtain the number of schizophrenic diagnoses divided by the number of schizophrenic *and* neurotic diagnoses. The minimum number of "calls" on which this figure was based was 214. *The figure ranged from 59% to 93%*. That is, at one hospital slightly over two out of every five calls was neurotic, while at the other extreme, there was a hospital where a call of neurotic occurred a little less frequently than once out of every 14 opportunities. It is interesting, however, to note the "validity" of this type of diagnostic distinction. The proportion of schizophrenic diagnostic calls *on admission* at 30 hospitals averaged 76.1% with a standard deviation of 8.57%. However, the proportion of functional psychotic to functional psychotics *and* other neuropsychiatric disorders (excluding neurological disorders, but including personality as well as neurotic disorders) *remaining* in the hospital was 95.1% with a standard deviation of 2.81% for the 30 hospitals as of October 31, 1959, and an average of 93.1% with a standard deviation of 3.08% as of October 31, 1960. The neurotics did have a considerably greater expectation of release than the schizophrenics, being roughly one to four in the admission group, but one to twenty in the resident population on a given day.

A first set of testable hypotheses deals with whether the proportion of calls which were schizophrenic was associated with hospital characteristics such as size and staffing. The correlation between the proportion of schizophrenic diagnostic calls and hospital size was random, .01. The correlation between the proportion of schizophrenic calls and staffing per patient was also statistically insignificant, .11.

A second set of hypotheses dealt with the correlation between the proportion of schizophrenic calls and the criterion measures of effectiveness. The correlation between proportion of schizophrenic diagnoses and the intake per size measure was —.14, which was statistically insignificant. Given the particular correlations obtained, when the proportion of schizophrenic diagnoses was held constant by means of partial correlation, the correlation between intake per size and staffing *increased* slightly rather than decreased.

The next hypothesis to be tested dealt with geographical location. The correlation between proportion of schizophrenic diagnoses and rural–urban location was —.18 which with 30 cases is statistically insignificant. Given the particular numerical assignment (numerically high values being rural, numerically low values being urban), whatever trend there might have been was for rural hospitals to make a higher proportion of neurotic calls than urban hospitals.

The final area of investigation was the correlation between the proportion of schizophrenic calls and the two major criteria of effectiveness, FSR and percentage of men with two or more years' continuous residence, % 2+ years. The correlation between the proportion of men called schizophrenic and percentage of early FSR was —.51. This correlation was statistically significant, but it was in a direction opposite to the one most readily predicted. That is, *hospitals where calls of schizophrenic were relatively less frequent had significantly higher percentages of early FSR.* This was surprising because the expectation was that neurotics have more favorable prognoses than schizophrenics. A hospital could conceivably have achieved a high early FSR score by diagnosing a relatively high number of neurotics as schizophrenic, thus including a disproportionate number of easier cases in the "schizophrenic" group. The opposite was what did in fact occur, a matter which increases the confidence which may be placed in the significant correlation between size and FSR. Another way in which this point can be made is that *if the measure of proportion of schizophrenic calls is held constant by partial correlation, the correlation between size and FSR increases from —.37 to —.42.*

The correlation between the proportion of diagnoses which were schizophrenic and the percentage of men with two or more years hospitalization was .33. This correlation borders on statistical significance (critical ratio equals 1.93) and is in the direction of hospitals with a high percentage of men with long residence being associated with a high proportion of schizophrenic diagnoses. However, because the proportion of schizophrenic diagnoses is minimally and positively associated with staffing (i.e. .11), *when the proportion of schizophrenic diagnoses is held constant by means of partial correlation, the correlation between staffing and percentage of men with two or more years' hospitalization increases, from —.73 to —.81.* In short, as with other computations in this section, investigation of the proportion of schizophrenic diagnoses increases rather than decreases our confidence in the associations between the criteria of effectiveness and the hospital characteristics of size and staffing.

While the purpose of investigating the proportion of schizophrenic diagnoses was to deal with a potential source of error in the criterion variables, the finding of the significant negative correlation between the proportion of schizophrenic diagnoses and percentage of early FSR was challenging. A large number of additional analyses were completed in order to find some third variable which when held constant would reduce the correlation between early FSR and proportion of schizophrenic diagnoses below the level of significance. No reasonable hypothesis was found which, when tested, led to an explanation of the finding. It is always reasonable and proper with inductive work to presume that there was a failure to formulate the proper hypothesis or to obtain a measure of the relevant variable. However, after running through a fair number of variables it seems the best explanation of the finding is that it illustrates the view presented by Cumming and Cumming (1957) cited in Chapter 4 and concepts such as those expressed by Menninger (1964):

> Words like "schizophrenia" and "manic-depressive" and "psychotic," for example, frighten patients and worry their anxious relatives and friends. The use of these alarming terms also affects us psychiatrists. They lead us back into the pessimism and helplessness of the days when mental illness was thought to be made up of many specific "diseases," and when each "disease" bore a formidable label and a gloomy prognosis. . . .
>
> . . . these technical words have become pejorative. They no longer mean merely psychiatric illness; they mean something despised. . . .
>
> To sum up, I think many words psychiatrists use are dangerous. They

misrepresent mental illness and permit the public and even psychiatrists to entertain a pessimistic view of mental illness.

The widespread pessimism about mental illness may explain why so little is done about it.

## SUMMARY

In this chapter we have tested the association of the hospital characteristics of size and staffing with measures of hospital effectiveness. Because 30 hospitals were used, it was possible to compute partial correlations which permitted the evaluation of one hospital characteristic (size *or* staffing) with the other held constant. When this was done, it was found that both size and staffing have demonstrable value, and the particular beneficial impact each has is on different measures of hospital effectiveness. Finally, additional analyses were performed to take into account possible alternative explanations for the obtained results. The effect of these analyses was to increase rather than reduce the confidence which may be put in the findings indicating the beneficial effects of small size and high staffing.

## CHAPTER 7

# *Hospital Characteristics Associated with Effectiveness*

IN THE foregoing material we have indicated that both size and staffing were significantly associated with measures of effectiveness, but that these characteristics might well have different areas of impact. The present section will refine the previous work by investigating some 27 hospital characteristics.[1] Some of these characteristics will deal with the relative staffing of particular professions, some will deal with the relative amounts of money spent in particular areas of hospital endeavor, and some will deal with special programs and miscellaneous hospital characteristics.

In working with this material, two measures of effectiveness will be used. The first will be a measure of rapid release, FSR, the percentage of patients achieving an early first significant release at each hospital. As noted previously, the FSR measure which will be used will be the one corrected for age and marital statuses. The second measure will be the percentage of patients at each hospital with two or more years' continuous hospitalization. The measures of turnover previously used were all intercorrelated over .80 with each other, and over .70 with each other even when FSR had been held constant by partial correlation.

Of the three measures of turnover, percentage of patients with long hospital residence was selected for the present work because it had the highest correlation with the other two measures, and because the sampling on which it was based was both broader and more systematic than that of the other two measures of turnover. Finally, this variable is the one that most directly measures the "second," chronic, static hospital noted by Jones and Sidebotham (1962).

[1] Details of the test–retest correlation for successive time periods and the means and ranges for these measures will be found in Appendix 3 of this book.

Data dealing with expenditure and staffing were obtained from the VA *monthly Field Station Summary*. Because the language of these reports is specialized and the number of variables dealt with is large, the variables, intercorrelations, and discussions will be presented in a sequence of separate areas of interest. Two general points need to be made. The first is that the measure called *%-psychiatric* will be introduced in many of the statistical analyses. Even with the present sample in which the average hospital had psychiatric patients as 96.5% of its average daily patient load, %-psychiatric was highly stable over time and significantly associated (—.46) with the number of employees per patient. A second general point is that at times the data will be in terms of *per diem* or cost per patient per day, and at other times the data will be in terms of *staffing* or employees per patient. The use of one or the other of these bases was determined by the manner in which data were reported in the *VA Field Station Summary*. However, overall *per diem* and overall staffing were practically identical, the correlation between the two for the 30 hospitals in this study being .95.

## THE STRATEGY AND PRESENTATION OF STATISTICAL ANALYSES

Tables 10 through 15, which present the findings of this part of the investigation, all follow the same form. On the left-hand side of the table are presented the hospital characteristics of staffing or expense under investigation. The first five columns, from left to right, present the correlations between these characteristics and (a) some measure of overall expense or staffing; (b) the criterion of percentage of patients achieving an early (FSR) release; (c) the criterion of the percentage of patients with long (two or more years continuous) hospital residence; (d) size of hospital; and, (e) per cent of patient load devoted to psychiatric cases. The focus of interest is on the correlations between hospital characteristics such as expense and the two criteria of effectiveness. However, correlations do not indicate causation, and more important for the strategy of data analysis, a correlation between two variables may be the result of a third variable. This is the reason for presenting correlations between expense variables and size of hospitals and %-psychiatric. Size was significantly associated[1] with percentage of early release (—.37), percentage of patients with long residence (.51), and with number of full time employees per patient (—.44). While the %-psychiatric measure was randomly associated with size (—.06), percentage of early release (.06), and percentage of patients with long residence (.12), it was significantly correlated with many expense variables. For example, the correlation between %-psychiatric and full time employees per patient was —.46 while the correlation between %-psychiatric and physicians per patient was —.58. As such, size and %-psychiatric are variables which need to be held constant by double-partial correlation (McNemar, 1962, pp. 164–7) so that the association between measures of expense and measures of efficiency can be presented without the influence of size of hospital and expense for general medical cases. The last or right-hand three columns of each of these six tables present such double-partial correlations. These three columns present from left to right (f) the correlation of the hospital characteristic to a measure of expense (for example, number of treatment personnel per patient) with both size and %-psychiatric held constant; (g) the correlation between the expense variable and percentage of early release with both size and %-psychiatric held constant; and (h) the correlation between the expense variable and percentage of patients with long hospital residence with both size and %-psychiatric held constant. These last two columns represent the key findings of this study.

A final note on strategy is necessary. When dealing with "raw" expenses such as cost per patient per day (*per diem*) or number of staff per patient, the measures in the different areas (for example, administration vs. nursing) were highly correlated. In this case, the third column from the right (column f) will show highly significant correlations even after size and %-psychiatric have been held constant. A general expense factor is indicated by such findings, and percentages were used to decrease it while investigating the relative effects of specific sub-areas of expense. The degree to which this procedure was successful will be indicated by column f, the correlation between the particular (percentage) expense variable and the

[1] In all the tables, for the first five columns, correlations of .36 are significant at the .05 level ($z$=1.96); correlations of .46 are significant at the .01 level ($z$=2.56); and correlations of .56 are significant at the .001 level ($z$=3.30). For double-partial correlations, because of the loss of two degrees of freedom, the correlations required for the respective levels of significance are .37, .47, and .58.

TABLE 10. *Correlations for 30 psychiatric hospitals between criteria of effectiveness and amount spent and percentage of total amount spent in four basic areas*

| Expense variable | Total *per diem* (a) | %-early release (b) | %-long residence (c) | Size (d) | %-psy-chiatric (e) | With size and %-psychiatric constant: Total *per diem* (f) | With size and %-psychiatric constant: %-early release (g) | With size and %-psychiatric constant: %-long residence (h) |
|---|---|---|---|---|---|---|---|---|
| General administration (GA) | .91 | .39 | −.72 | −.69 | −.36 | .86 | .28 | −.54 |
| Non-nursing patient care (NNPC) | .94 | .18 | −.68 | −.43 | −.56 | .88 | .07 | −.64 |
| Nursing care (NC) | .87 | .24 | −.71 | −.47 | −.32 | .81 | .11 | −.61 |
| Food and shelter (F & S) | .85 | −.06 | −.34 | −.29 | −.47 | .78 | −.25 | −.17 |
| % for GA | .25 | .57 | −.41 | −.67 | .06 | −.14 | .47 | −.10 |
| % for NNPC | .56 | .18 | −.50 | −.21 | −.49 | .33 | .11 | −.44 |
| % for NC | −.22 | .14 | −.10 | .03 | .29 | −.08 | .16 | −.09 |
| % for F & S | −.30 | −.48 | .59 | .39 | .04 | −.11 | −.39 | .49 |

overall, more general expense variable with size and %-psychiatric held constant. For example, in Table 10, the top four rows deal with raw *per diem* figures and the correlations in column f are highly significant. This led to the use of percentage of the total *per diem* expense in the four areas (the bottom four rows) and in column f the correlations were all statistically insignificant, indicating the success of this statistical procedure.

## HOSPITAL EFFECTIVENESS AND *PER DIEM* EXPENSE IN FOUR BASIC AREAS

The allocation of funds for VA psychiatric hospitals may be broken down into four major areas: (a) administration (including the Hospital Director's Office and Personnel, Supply, Registrar, and Fiscal Divisions); (b) non-nursing patient care (including all professional treatment staff other than nurses); (c) nursing care (nurses and nursing assistants); and, (d) food and shelter (including Housekeeping, Engineering, and Dietetics). Across all hospitals in the sample, the first area, administration, accounted for approximately 10% of the *per diem* expense, while the other three areas accounted for roughly equal amounts of the remaining 90%.

The first four rows of Table 10 present the correlations between *per diem* expense in each of the four areas and the eight measures (columns) discussed in the immediately preceding section. While each of the four areas of expense contributed to the total *per diem*, it is interesting to note the extent to which the correlations between each area and total *per diem* was (a) very high, and, (b) of essentially equal magnitude. That is, across 30 hospitals whose range of overall *per diem* during the study period was from $10.19 to $17.67, the more money that was available, the more money was spent in all four areas. Ideally, it would be expected that there would be a stable amount of money needed per patient per day in an area such as food and shelter, particularly when variables such as size and %-psychiatric had been held constant. Similarly, it would be expected, under ideal conditions, that as the amount of money available per patient increased, an increasingly disproportionate amount of this money would be spent on patient care. The correlations presented in Table 10 indicate that this ideal allocation of funds was not achieved to any overwhelming extent, but rather, as Parkinson (1960) stated in his second law, it seems that "expenditure rises to meet income."

A second matter of interest in Table 10 deals with the correlations between *per diem* expense in four areas and the two measures of hospital effectiveness. While the intercorrelations among *per diem* expenses in the four areas were high (the median being .75), there was some variation in the correlations between the expense in the four areas and the two measures of hospital effectiveness. For example, a relatively high *per diem* expense for administration was significantly associated with high early release while high expense for food and shelter was associated negatively, albeit insignificantly, with early release. Similarly, the association between expense for food and shelter and a low percentage of patients with long residence was markedly different from associations between this latter variable and expenses in the other three areas.

To evaluate more accurately the effect of increasing *per diem* in each of the four areas, it was necessary to exclude the general factor of total *per diem* as it influenced all four areas. The manner in which this was done was to determine the correlation between the measures of hospital effectiveness and the *percentage* of the total *per diem* spent in each of the four areas. The decision to use a percentage was based in part on a desire to avoid the loss of another degree of freedom involved in a further (triple) partial correlation. Second, the use of a percentage more closely approximated the hospital situation in which limited funds must be allocated, and in which, by chance, an increase in one area is associated with a decrease in some other area. This may be illustrated by the empirical finding that the median correlation for the intercorrelations among percentages of the *per diem* allocation spent in the four areas was —.39.

As overall *per diem* increased, the per cent of the *per diem* spent on nursing care (—.22) and food and shelter (—.30) tended to decrease, while the amount spent on administration (.25) and non-nursing patient care (.56) tended to increase. Only the last correlation, that between total *per diem* and percentage of *per diem* spent on (professional) non-nursing patient care was statistically significant. However, when size and %-psychiatric were held constant by means of double-partial correlation, the correlation between total *per diem* and percentage of *per diem* spent on non-nursing patient care declined to .33. This correlation, which bordered on but did not reach statistical significance ($z = 1.72$), supported the adequacy of the statistical procedure used to rule out the effects of general level of *per diem* expense. On an administrative level, it also indicated that there was a wide gap between practice and the ideal of increased funds being used disproportionately for patient care services.

There was a highly significant negative correlation (—.67) between size and percentage of *per diem* spent in the area of general administration. This finding was maintained even after total *per diem* was held constant by partial correlation (—.65) and also when *per diem* was measured in dollars and cents rather than as a percentage. In this latter case, the correlation between *per diem* expense of general administration services and size (with total *per diem* held constant by partial correlation) was —.65. In short, large hospitals were more efficient in terms of decreased *per capita* expense for administrative overhead.

The last two columns of Table 10 present the double-partial correlations between percentage of *per diem* spent in each of the four areas and the two measures of effectiveness with size of hospital and %-psychiatric held constant. There were three major findings. First, a relatively high percentage of *per diem* spent on administration was significantly associated with a high early release rate. The finding indicated that the more money spent on administrative services the higher the percentage of early release. Where data previously presented confirmed that as size increased administrative overhead decreased, the present material indicated that low expenditure in the administrative area may not necessarily have been a worthwhile saving. While the limits of the present research do not permit explanation of why greater expenditure in the administrative area was associated with higher early release, it is relevant to cite Ginzberg (1949, p. 327): "A good administrator needs good assistants. In addition, he must rely on operating statistics and accounting as instruments of control. . . . The most important challenge to the administrator is the development of methods to extend and improve team relations within the hospital so that scarce specialized personnel can be conserved."

A second major finding was the significant negative correlation between percentage of the *per diem* spent on (professional) non-nursing patient care and percentage of patients with long hospital residence. It is important to note that just as in previous research small size was associated with early release and high staffing with low percentage of long-residence patients, in the present study high percentage of *per diem* spent on administration was associated with early release while high percentage of *per diem* spent on non-nursing patient care was associated with low percentage of patients with long hospitalization. These latter results were obtained in a situation which held constant size and overall staffing.

A third and final point was the significantly unfavorable association of percentage of *per diem* spent on food and shelter with both measures of hospital effectiveness. In short, relatively higher expenses for food and shelter were associated with lower percentage of early release (—.39) and higher percentage of patients with long residence (.49). Again, the statistical analysis ruled out interpretations based on concepts of different hospital size, hospital mission, or amount of overall *per diem*.

## HOSPITAL EFFECTIVENESS AND TREATMENT PERSONNEL

This section is analogous to the previous one save that the variables deal with full time employees per patient rather than dollar cost. The focus is on staffing per patient of physicians, psychologists, social workers, physical medicine and rehabilitation (PMR) workers, nurses, and nursing assistants. These six groups are the ones which are the largest numerically and, in the vast majority of cases, the most important ones in the treatment of psychiatric patients.[1]

One procedural point needs to be made: "all" staff (e.g. Table 11) will refer to the number of all (including administrative and food and shelter) employees per patient while "treatment" staff (e.g. Table 12) will refer to the sum of psychiatrists, psychologists, social workers, PMR workers, nurses, and nursing assistants per patient.

In many ways, the data presented in the first five columns of Table 11 parallel the previous findings dealing with *per diem* expense. There was a general variable of staffing or expense which was manifested by the significant correlations between each staff group and total staff. This finding held even when size and %-psychiatric were held constant. Further, the matrix of intercorrelations between the six types of treatment personnel had a median correlation of .63.

[1] The present definition of treatment staff does not include such professional staff members as chaplains, dentists, and pharmacists who are important in function, but relatively few in number at each hospital.

TABLE 11. *Correlations for 30 psychiatric hospitals between criteria of effectiveness and staffing per patient for six groups of personnel*

| | | | | | | With size and %-psychiatric constant | | |
|---|---|---|---|---|---|---|---|---|
| Expense variable | All staff | %-early release | %-long residence | Size | %-psy-chiatric | All staff | %-early release | %-long residence |
| All treatment staff | .93 | .20 | −.75 | −.52 | −.33 | .90 | .02 | −.66 |
| Physicians | .60 | .29 | −.46 | −.13 | −.58 | .49 | .33 | −.45 |
| Psychologists | .73 | .14 | −.60 | −.41 | −.44 | .58 | .01 | −.48 |
| Social workers | .84 | .17 | −.66 | −.35 | −.47 | .77 | .08 | −.61 |
| PMR workers | .66 | .01 | −.59 | −.71 | −.09 | .53 | −.39 | −.36 |
| Nurses | .74 | .34 | −.66 | −.58 | −.29 | .59 | .20 | −.50 |
| Nursing assistants | .88 | .13 | −.68 | −.39 | −.25 | .84 | −.01 | −.59 |

All the measures of staff per patient for the six types of personnel were similar in being insignificantly associated with percentage of early release, while being significantly associated with a low percentage of patients with long hospital residence. In all cases the direction of association was for all types of treatment personnel to be lessened in large hospitals and in hospitals with a greater percentage of the patient load devoted to psychiatric cases.

The results of holding size and %-psychiatric constant by means of double-partial correlation are presented in the last three columns of Table 11. Of particular interest was that number of PMR workers per patient was significantly and negatively correlated with a high percentage of early release. High staffing per patient of all six groups of personnel was significantly associated with a low percentage of patients with long hospital residence, even after size and %-psychiatric had been held constant. In short, Table 11 indicates that high professional staffing was significantly associated with turnover. However, Table 11 also indicates that there was a general staffing variable which must be taken into consideration before it becomes possible to evaluate the differential contribution of specific treatment groups.

Table 12 parallels the last four rows of Table 10 in that a percentage was used to reduce the effect of the general expense or staffing variable. The base for the percentage figures in Table 12 was the number of treatment personnel. As the total number of treatment staff increased, the percentages of registered nurses, social workers, and psychologists tended to increase while the percentages of nursing assistants and PMR workers tended to decrease. In similar fashion, as the %-psychiatric increased, the percentage of treatment staff represented by physicians, social workers, and psychologists decreased.

As is the case throughout, the key data is in the last three columns which present correlations with size and %-psychiatric held constant. With the exception of the PMR variable, the use of a percentage and the partialling of the effects of size and %-psychiatric effectively reduced the correlation between total treatment staff and the percentage of treatment staff represented by each specific personnel group. The correlation between percentage of treatment staff who were physicians and percentage of early release approached very closely but did not reach statistical significance. The greater the percentage of treatment staff who were social workers, the lower was

TABLE 12. *Correlations for 30 psychiatric hospitals between criteria of effectiveness and percentage of treatment staff accounted for by six groups of personnel*

| Percentage of treatment staff | All treatment staff | %-early release | %-long residence | Size | %-psychiatric | With size and %-psychiatric held constant | | |
|---|---|---|---|---|---|---|---|---|
| | | | | | | All treatment staff | %-early release | %-long residence |
| Physicians | −.03 | .21 | −.04 | .19 | −.44 | −.13 | .36 | −.10 |
| Psychologists | .35 | .10 | −.40 | −.27 | −.36 | .11 | .02 | −.28 |
| Social workers | .43 | .12 | −.44 | −.17 | −.41 | .28 | .09 | −.39 |
| PMR workers | −.32 | −.31 | .21 | −.26 | .30 | −.50 | −.49 | .38 |
| Nurses | .45 | .39 | −.32 | −.51 | −.12 | .20 | .26 | −.05 |
| Nursing assistants | −.33 | −.30 | .33 | .52 | .24 | .06 | −.16 | .03 |

the percentage of patients with long hospital residence. In the present analysis, the percentages of psychologists, nurses, and nursing assistants, were not significantly associated with either early release or long hospitalization.

The percentage of treatment staff who were PMR workers required a different statistical analysis because of the significant negative correlation between this measure and overall size of treatment staff. The procedure used was to substitute overall treatment staff for %-psychiatric as the second variable to be held constant by double-partial correlation.[1] When this was done, the correlation between percentage of treatment staff who were PMR workers and percentage of patients with long hospital residence was .08. In short, the significant (.38) correlation between high percentage of PMR workers and long residence was a function of the percentage of PMR workers increasing when the total treatment staff decreased. However, holding size and overall staffing constant, the correlation between percentage of treatment staff who were PMR workers and percentage of early release was —.54, a highly significant correlation indicative of a negative association between percentage of early release and percentage of treatment staff who were PMR workers.

Combining the results presented in Tables 11 and 12, it may be said that (a) high patient-care staffing was significantly associated with decreased percentage of patients with long hospital residence, but (b) in general there was no group of personnel with particular effectiveness, save (c) a high percentage of physicians and low percentage of PMR workers in terms of early release, and a high percentage of social workers in terms of long residence.

[1] While size was significantly correlated with the criterion measures of effectiveness and could not be dropped from the partial correlation analysis, %-psychiatric was randomly correlated with early release, long residence, and size. There usually was a significant correlation between %-psychiatric and the staffing or expense variable, but percentage of treatment staff who were PMR workers was insignificantly correlated with %-psychiatric and the substitution of overall treatment staff per patient in place of %-psychiatric was possible. However, the simplification of variables to be held constant made a second procedure possible: holding size and overall treatment staff constant by double-partial correlation, the correlation between PMR workers per patient and percentage of early release was —.48 (significant at the .01 level), while the correlation between number of PMR workers per patient and percentage of patients with long hospital residence was .03 (statistically insignificant). That is, the same statistical decisions were obtained by both strategies.

## THE ASSOCIATION OF OTHER HOSPITAL CHARACTERISTICS AND EFFECTIVENESS

This section will present data concerning miscellaneous hospital characteristics. The first two of these characteristics deal with the training function of the hospital, specifically the presence or absence of a psychiatric resident program and the relative size of the psychology trainee program. While training is a valuable thing in itself and does not have patient release as a prime goal, it is interesting, as may be seen in Table 13, that both training programs were significantly associated with a low percentage of patients with long hospital residence. These findings were obtained after size and %-psychiatric had been held constant and after there was evidence that size of total treatment staff was not significantly associated with the two training programs. As with training, a research program has a long-term rather than an immediate goal. While a research program may stimulate staff members and help in the recruitment of professional staff, the presence of a large research program was not significantly associated with either of the two measures of hospital effectiveness after size and %-psychiatric had been held constant. The next hospital characteristic investigated was the size of family care program. A large family care program was randomly associated with early release, but very significantly associated with a low percentage of patients with long residence, even after size and %-psychiatric had been held constant by partial correlation. As other research (Ullmann and Berkman, 1959a, b, c; Ullmann, Berkman and Hamister, 1958; Giovannoni and Ullmann, 1961) has indicated, family care is generally an effective program and has a particular value for men with long hospitalization who are placed from poor prognosis wards. It is this specific group that is central to the percentage of patients with two or more years' continuous residence. The variable of rural–urban hospital location is frequently discussed today, and it is generally thought that an isolated, rural setting militates against obtaining high release rates. This concept was not supported by the present findings. However, what was found when the intercorrelations among hospital characteristics were studied, was that the rural–urban variable was significantly associated with measures which make a hospital "more modern." The more rural the hospitals the fewer were the physicians (—.55), psychologists (—.54), and social workers (—.39) per patient. Also the more rural

TABLE 13. *Correlations for 30 psychiatric hospitals between criteria of effectiveness and various hospital characteristics*

| Variables | All treatment staff | %-early release | %-long residence | Size | %-psychiatric | With size and %-psychiatric held constant: All treatment staff | %-early release | %-long residence |
|---|---|---|---|---|---|---|---|---|
| Residency program | .20 | .07 | −.18 | .29 | −.56 | .25 | .27 | −.43 |
| Psychology trainees | .39 | .31 | −.54 | −.41 | −.26 | .11 | .21 | −.41 |
| Research program | .23 | .30 | −.30 | −.35 | −.35 | −.13 | .23 | −.09 |
| Family care program | .46 | .12 | −.62 | −.32 | −.08 | .35 | .01 | −.55 |
| Rural–urban location | −.20 | .09 | .06 | −.35 | .45 | −.36 | −.07 | .25 |
| Applicants per size | .40 | .46 | −.54 | −.14 | −.13 | .36 | .45 | −.54 |
| Medication | .71 | .27 | −.68 | −.51 | −.34 | .51 | .13 | −.55 |
| Volunteers | .31 | −.19 | −.14 | −.26 | −.46 | .02 | −.34 | .01 |

hospitals were significantly less likely to have a psychiatric resident program (—.66) or a large research program (—.36). To quote Ginzberg (1949, p. 277), "To the maximum extent possible, the State should expand its beds in large urban centers because of the greater ease of securing personnel in large communities." The present findings agree with this statement, particularly in terms of the professional staff and the research and training characteristics that attract professional staff, and support the building of hospitals in urban areas on the basis of staff recruitment rather than patient release.

Another characteristic studied was the number of applications for hospitalization received divided by the average daily patient load, i.e. applications per size. *The higher the number of applications per size, the more favorable were both the measures of early release and long residence.*[1] The correlation between applications per size and rural–urban setting was random (—.02) indicating that this variable was not influenced by geographical location. Applications per size will figure importantly in our discussions of results in Part III of this book, and the direction of our remarks is foreshadowed in the following sentences by Cumming and Cumming (1957, p. 68): "It is well recognized that the decision to discharge a patient is related to the question of how badly his bed is needed. Since most hospitals are somewhat crowded, what constitutes sufficient overcrowding to exert a 'statistical pressure' toward discharge?"

Two additional characteristics are presented below a line which separates them from the remainder of Table 13. This line emphasizes that complete data for these variables were not available. Because of the attention these variables have received in the literature, the information which was collected will be presented. The first additional variable is that of cost of drugs per patient per day. The data were defective in that information was not available for one of the

[1] The double-partial correlations of .36 between treatment staff per patient and family care and applications per size were so close to statistical significance and the variables so important in terms of effectiveness that further computations were carried out. Because neither family care nor applications per size were significantly associated with %-psychiatric, treatment staff per patient was substituted for %-psychiatric. The double-partial correlations which held size and treatment staff constant led to .00 and —.46 correlations between family care and percentage early release and percentage long hospital residence, respectively, and .48 and —.43 between applications per size and percentage early release and percentage long hospital residence, respectively.

hospitals for one of the two years under study. The correlation for 29 hospitals between *per diem* cost of drugs for successive years was .92. For the present work, the *per diem* cost of drugs during the single year for which information was available for all 30 hospitals was used. The range of *per diem* cost for drugs was from $.09 to $.42 with an average of $.198. From Table 13, the reader will note that even after holding size and %-psychiatric constant, the cost of drugs was significantly correlated with size of treatment staff. That is, the more treatment personnel there were per patient, the greater was the amount of money spent on patients' medication. Because the correlation between cost of medication and %-psychiatric was random, the measure of treatment staff per patient was substituted for %-psychiatric in the double-partial correlation. With size and treatment staff held constant, the correlation between medication and long hospital residence approached, but did not reach statistical significance, —.32. With size and treatment staff held constant, the correlation between medication and early release was insignificant, —.09.

The final hospital characteristic investigated was number of regularly scheduled volunteer hours per patient. Data were available for only 29 of the 30 hospitals. The correlation between number of regularly scheduled volunteer hours during the two successive years of this study was .95. The range of number of regularly scheduled volunteer hours per patient per year was from 6 to 60 with an average of 22. The correlations reported in Table 13 indicate that the number of volunteer hours per patient approached but did not reach statistical significance in a manner indicative of a high number of volunteer hours being associated with a low rate of early release. The present results do not support and may even, on the surface, appear to contradict the recommendation of the Joint Commission on Mental Illness and Health (1961, p. 253) that "Volunteer work with mental hospital patients done by college students and many others should be encouraged and extended." It should be noted that the work cited by the Joint Commission on Mental Illness and Health (1961, pp. 88–93) was accomplished under close professional supervision as a new program centered on patients with prolonged hospitalization. The members of these programs were college students who had as their orientation the problem of "how to develop a relationship that would work toward the patient's recovery" (Joint Commission on Mental Illness and Health, 1961, p. 91). The typical VA volunteer[1] differs in education, supervision, program, and orientation from those described by the Joint Commission. Only three per cent of all VA volunteers were enrolled in any type of school or college and half were between 45 and 65 years of age.

## A FURTHER ANALYSIS OF ADMINISTRATIVE EXPENSES

As may have been noted from Table 10 and our discussion thereof, the percentage of the total *per diem* devoted to the area of general administration was highly correlated (.47) with percentage of early release even after size and %-psychiatric had been held constant by double-partial correlation. Further, the correlation between early release and size was insignificant (.02) when percentage of *per diem* spent on general administration was held constant. In short, the area of general administration was of import in itself and as a lead to more definite determination of the correlates of hospital characteristics that are of particular value.

The area of general administration may be broken down into five sub-areas: the office of the manager, registrar, fiscal, personnel, and supply. Table 14 is analogous to Table 10 in the information presented. The first five rows of Table 14 deal with the *per diem* expenditure for each of the five sub-areas, while the second five rows of Table 14 deal with the percentage of the total *per diem* devoted to each of the five areas.

The material presented in Table 14 parallels the material in Table 10 in that the direct measures of expenditure in sub-areas are highly associated with total expenditure, the only exception being the office of the manager. The obtained correlations with criterion measures of effectiveness might well be a function of the overlap with total *per diem*, and hence the major emphasis needs to be on the second five rows in which a percentage of the *per diem* is used to rule out the effects of total *per diem*. When this was done and size and %-psychiatric were held constant by double-partial correlation, some very interesting findings were obtained. The major one was the

[1] Anonymous. Recruitment and retention of volunteers in Veterans Administration Voluntary Service. *VA Field Station Summary*, April, 1960, pp. 72–77. Washington, D.C.: Department of Medicine and Surgery, Veterans Administration.

TABLE 14. *Correlations for 30 psychiatric hospitals between criteria of effectiveness and amount spent and percentage of total amount spent in five sub-areas of general administration*

| Expense variable | Total *per diem* | %-early release | %-long residence | Size | %-psy-chiatric | With size and %-psychiatric held constant: Total *per diem* | %-early release | %-long residence |
|---|---|---|---|---|---|---|---|---|
| Manager's office | .48 | .38 | −.54 | −.85 | −.08 | −.04 | .15 | −.20 |
| Registrar | .87 | .36 | −.70 | −.35 | −.53 | .76 | .36 | −.69 |
| Fiscal | .72 | .41 | −.67 | −.86 | −.10 | .63 | .22 | −.51 |
| Personnel | .88 | .06 | −.52 | −.54 | −.45 | .75 | −.19 | −.30 |
| Supply | .69 | .23 | −.53 | −.87 | −.06 | .59 | −.20 | −.17 |
| % for manager | .31 | .39 | −.31 | −.84 | .17 | −.13 | .15 | .22 |
| % for registrar | .11 | .44 | −.29 | .12 | −.24 | .07 | .55 | −.39 |
| % for fiscal | .13 | .43 | −.36 | −.77 | .25 | −.36 | .24 | .00 |
| % for personnel | .35 | −.10 | −.09 | −.37 | −.20 | .08 | −.27 | .17 |
| % for supply | .01 | .20 | −.11 | −.74 | .40 | −.44 | −.17 | .44 |

significant correlation between effectiveness and the percentage of the *per diem* devoted to the registrar sub-area. The greater the relative investment in registrar, the higher was the percentage of early release (.55) and the lower the percentage of patients with long residence (—.39). In none of the four other sub-areas did the correlations approach this degree of favorable association with the measures of effectiveness. In fact, there was a trend for percentage of the *per diem* devoted to the personnel office to be negatively associated with percentage of early release and for the percentage of the *per diem* devoted to the supply office to be positively associated with a high percentage of patients with long residence. The significant correlation between percentage of *per diem* devoted to supply and percentage of patients with long hospitalization was a result of the negative correlation between percentage of the *per diem* devoted to supply and total *per diem*. When total *per diem* was substituted for %-psychiatric in double-partial correlations (the second variable held constant being size) the correlation between absolute and relative amounts of expenditure on supply and percentage of patients with long residence became insignificant (.19 and .18 respectively). This explanation, however, does not hold for the negative correlation between percentage of the total *per diem* devoted to personnel and the effectiveness criterion of percentage of patients with early release. In short, the focal element in the area of general administration would clearly seem to be the sort of services rendered by the registrar's office in comparison with the functions of the personnel office. This matter will be returned to in the third part of this book.

## A FURTHER ANALYSIS OF "FOOD AND SHELTER" EXPENSES

Just as the area of general administration seemed to be favorably associated with early release so the area of "food and shelter" was unfavorably associated with both measures of effectiveness (cf. the last line of Table 10, columns g and h). The area called "food and shelter" may be divided into money spent on dietetics, engineering, and housekeeping. Table 15 follows the form of Table 10 in presenting the absolute and relative amounts of the total *per diem* devoted to these three sub-areas.

TABLE 15. *Correlations for 30 psychiatric hospitals between criteria of effectiveness and amount spent and percentage of total amount spent in three sub-areas: dietetics, engineering, and housekeeping*

| | | | | | | With size and %-psychiatric constant | | |
|---|---|---|---|---|---|---|---|---|
| | Total *per diem* | %-early release | %-long residence | Size | %-psychiatric | Total *per diem* | %-early release | %-long residence |
| Dietetics | .68 | −.10 | −.30 | −.08 | −.35 | .71 | −.13 | −.26 |
| Engineering | .75 | −.02 | −.24 | −.35 | −.41 | .61 | −.17 | −.05 |
| Housekeeping | .68 | −.11 | −.38 | −.26 | −.41 | .55 | −.24 | −.25 |
| % for dietetics | −.68 | −.35 | .60 | .69 | .30 | −.35 | −.18 | .36 |
| % for engineering | .00 | −.22 | .39 | .04 | −.08 | −.03 | −.22 | .45 |
| % for housekeeping | .24 | −.28 | −.06 | −.05 | −.21 | .16 | −.32 | .00 |

As with the other tables in this series, the information in Table 15 indicates that even with size and %-psychiatric held constant, as the total *per diem* increased, the amount spent in each sub-area increased. There was a general, but insignificant, trend for high expenditure in these areas to be unfavorably associated with the criterion measures of effectiveness, the only clearly significant correlation being that between a relatively high percentage of the total *per diem* accounted for by engineering and a high percentage of patients with long residence.

## MULTIPLE CORRELATIONS FOR STATISTICAL SUMMATION

It is reasonable to ask the extent to which and from what characteristics hospital effectiveness can be predicted. Of the 27 variables investigated (prior to analyses of sub-areas of administration and "food and shelter"), 17 were significantly correlated with percentage of long hospital residence even after size and %-psychiatric had been held constant by double-partial correlation. There was a multiple correlation of .862, after correction for shrinkage (McNemar, 1962, 169–87) between long hospital residence and three variables (number of treatment personnel per patient, size of family care program, and percentage of patients obtaining an early release). *If hospital size had been added as a fourth variable, the prediction would not have been increased.* The measure of percentage of early release was introduced here because logically a high early release rate reduces the number of patients who will, by chance, have long hospital residence.

There was a multiple correlation of .615 (after correction for shrinkage) between percentage of early release and three variables (percentage of *per diem* spent on general administration, percentage of *per diem* spent on "food and shelter," and number of applications per size). *Again, the addition of size would not have increased the correlation.* Finally, the variables which had been used to predict long hospital residence were specifically *not* used to derive the multiple correlation for the early release criterion.

A multiple correlation of .593 for long hospitalization can be obtained from percentage of *per diem* spent on general administration and applications per size. This compares favorably with the —.49 correlation between early release and long residence and can be substituted for early release in the prediction of percentage of patients with long hospitalization. When this substitution was made, the multiple correlation between percentage of patients with long hospital residence and four variables (number treatment staff per patient, home care program, amount of *per diem* spent on general administration, and applications per size) was .853 after correction for shrinkage. Aside from reducing the number of key variables, this procedure eliminated early release, a variable which could be manipulated administratively only through indirect means, from the equation accounting for long hospital residence.

## A SUMMARY TABULAR PRESENTATION

Table 16 repeats in layout and intent Table 9, but adds information gained from the analysis of hospital characteristics beyond size. Small size is included as one of the four characteristics helping to define "good" hospitals, because (a) in using a "high–low" designation, improper weight would otherwise be given to percentage of total *per diem* accounted for by general administration, and (b) to indicate what the analyses in Tables 10 through 13 *added* to size alone. The three additional variables (percentages of total *per diem* accounted for by general administration and by "food and shelter," and number of applications per size) were dichotomized. Of the 13 "poor" hospitals, eight had none of the four favorable indicators while five had one of the four favorable "signs." The reader may note that the material presented may be considered nine replications with different populations (defined by age and marital status). Eight of these nine replications yielded differences significant beyond the .05 level with two-tail test. Two additional points are worth noting: material in the additional analyses of Tables 14 and 15 was *not* used and the three characteristics are ones that can be manipulated (e.g. how money will be allocated within the hospital) with relative ease administratively.

The 17 "good" hospitals have a total size (ADPL) of 20,518 patients while the 13 "poor" hospitals have a total size of 23,059 patients. However, the "good" hospitals served 4202 admissions while the "poor" hospitals served 3010 admissions. That is, the "good" hospitals accounted for 47.1% of the ADPL while accounting for 58.3% of the admission population. While it would be

TABLE 16. *Comparison of "good" hospitals (at least two of the following four: small size, high percentage of* per diem *for general administrative, low percentage of* per diem *for food and shelter, high number of applications per size) with "poor" hospitals (i.e., none or at most one of the foregoing characteristics)*

| | 17 "good" hospitals | | 13 "poor" hospitals | | Differences | |
|---|---|---|---|---|---|---|
| | No. cases | % early FSR | No. cases | % early FSR | % early FSR | $X^2$ |
| MARRIED, NOTIFY WIFE | | | | | | |
| Age 17–30 | 207 | 83.6 | 126 | 73.8 | 9.8 | 4.07 |
| Age 31–45 | 979 | 79.6 | 581 | 66.1 | 13.5 | 34.20 |
| Age 46–59 | 157 | 67.5 | 87 | 56.3 | 11.2 | 2.56 |
| MARRIED, NOTIFY OTHER THAN WIFE | | | | | | |
| Age 17–30 | 121 | 76.0 | 89 | 61.8 | 14.2 | 4.20 |
| Age 31–45 | 698 | 69.9 | 412 | 53.9 | 16.0 | 28.20 |
| Age 46–59 | 133 | 56.4 | 81 | 38.3 | 18.1 | 5.90 |
| NEVER MARRIED | | | | | | |
| Age 17–30 | 680 | 60.3 | 581 | 47.2 | 13.1 | 21.25 |
| Age 31–45 | 1059 | 52.3 | 889 | 38.7 | 13.6 | 35.52 |
| Age 46–59 | 168 | 52.4 | 164 | 26.8 | 25.6 | 21.57 |

dangerous to make too much of such computations, it is interesting that the "good" hospitals represented 4.88 beds per new admission while the "poor" hospitals represented 7.66 beds per admission. In short, Table 16 presents a "frequency of cases" summary of the multiple correlational material reported in the immediately preceding section and may have some merit for administrative decisions about the building of new hospitals or the allocation of funds in existing hospitals.

## SUMMARY

This chapter screened a number of hospital characteristics to provide leads for administrative decisions and the investigation of hospital functioning. From this work two major summary results were obtained. The first was the development of strong multiple correlations for both major criteria of hospital effectiveness utilizing five variables: a high percentage of the *per diem* spent on general administration (with later emphasis on the services provided by the registrar), a low percentage of the *per diem* spent for "food and shelter," a high number of new applications for admission, a high number of treatment personnel per patient, and a large family care program. These characteristics are within the realm of administrative manipulation, and with the exception of number of treatment personnel per patient, do not require drastically increased expenditure. The second result is related to this first finding: size of hospital by itself did not add to the strength of the multiple correlations based on these five foregoing characteristics. We will use these findings to go beyond the variables of size or total treatment staff per patient to circumstances and relationships within the institution. While size will be an important variable in the following chapters, as it was in our statistical analyses, we will try to formulate the functions emphasized at effective hospitals and the behaviors that militate against the aversive consequences of the traditional large, public mental hospital.

# PART III

## *Discussions*

## CHAPTER 8

# *The Major Empirical Findings*

In the first part of this book we sketched background and theoretical considerations for the empirical results which were presented in the second part. In this third and final part of the book, we will bring together theory and findings. The focus of this first discussion chapter will be the major empirical findings with the immediate goal of deriving a framework in which such results are a reasonable outcome.

The major hypotheses with which this study began were confirmed: both small size and high staff-patient ratio were significantly associated with criteria of effectiveness. An important finding, however, was that the major impact of size and staffing were with different measures of effectiveness. This differential correlation between hospital characteristics and measures of effectiveness was noted throughout the empirical results and is one of the most important findings of this study.

There were two areas of effectiveness. The first was a percentage of men released within 274 days after admission to remain in the non-hospital community at least 90 consecutive days. This measure, early FSR, has been called early release. The second measure was the percentage of men with two or more years' continuous hospitalization, %2+ years, and has been called long hospitalization. Because of the high correlations (even after early release was held constant by partial correlation) between long hospital residence and measures of turnover at both intake and exit, long hospitalization may also be considered a measure of turnover. Whatever the names, there were different correlations between these operationally defined measures and various hospital characteristics.

The first major finding presented in chapter seven, and one which influenced many of the statistical analyses, was the high correlation among all staffing per patient and *per diem* expense variables. A good example of this point and the one made in the foregoing two chapters is provided by the *per diem* cost of the Registrar and Personnel

Divisions. As may be noted from Table 14, the former was significantly and favorably associated with both measures of effectiveness while the latter was minimally to negatively associated with measures of effectiveness. The correlation between *per diem* spent on Registrar Division and *per diem* spent on Personnel Division was .71. Even with the measures of size and %-psychiatric held constant, the correlation between cost of Registrar and Personnel was .48 and significant at the .01 level.

Tables 10 through 15 investigate specific hospital characteristics. The findings embodied in these tables can be put as questions to focus the discussion:

A: Why should the percentage of the *per diem* devoted to general administration be favorably associated with early release but not long hospitalization, while the percentage spent for non-nursing patient care be favorably associated with the long hospitalization measure and not early release?

B: Why should the percentage of the *per diem* spent on food and shelter be negatively associated with both early release and long hospitalization after both size and %-psychiatric had been held constant?

C: Why should the percentage of the treatment staff devoted to social workers, and to an even greater extent, the size of the home care program, be favorably associated with the long hospitalization measure, while the proportion of the treatment staff devoted to physicians and nurses was randomly associated with this measure of effectiveness?

D: Given the immediately preceding question, why should the percentage of the treatment staff who were physicians be favorably associated, the percentage of social workers be randomly associated, and the percentage of PMR workers negatively associated with the early release measure of effectiveness?

E: Why were the psychiatric residency and psychology trainee programs so favorably associated with the long hospitalization measure?

F: Why was the measure of new applications received per unit size favorably associated with *both* the early release and long hospitalization (turnover) criteria?

## CHAPTER 9

# *The Hospital Context*

WE WANT to delineate the context of the obtained statistical relationships. In doing so, let us return to the concept with which we started this book, that, following Allport (1933), there is no such thing as an institution *per se*, but only the behavior and objectives of people working together. This thought has been put by Strauss *et al.* (1963, p.150): "A hospital can be visualized as a professional locale—a geographical site where persons drawn from different professions come together to carry out their respective purposes." We are dealing with the behavior of individual organisms and "the social situation is unique only in so far as other organisms mediate the reinforcements, punishments, or other important environmental effects" (Ferster, 1958, p. 102). The social situation defines the performances that will be reinforced by other people. The range of reinforced behavior is limited by the needs and expectations of the persons who control and provide the reinforcement of behavior. We shall therefore orient ourselves to the behaviors individuals in the organizational setting are likely to emit in terms of available reinforcement.

While this chapter will have five sections, the overall plan is to move from the system as a whole to the supervisor–employee relationship. The outline of the argument that will be proposed is that the major consideration in funding hospitals fosters a custodial rather than treatment orientation. Without adherence to the major purpose of returning patients to the community, other behaviors come to be foci for reinforcement. This situation is intensified because the model used in hospitals is a bureaucratic one which is inappropriate to the task to be accomplished. This situation is likely to foster false personalization, good interpersonal relations, and an exchange or negotiated system.

This chapter will rely in great measure on the writings of other authors. I hope that this procedure will make it clear that the Veterans Administration hospitals at the time of the study were not unique but shared problems common to many large organizations.

## FUNDING AND DISPLACEMENT OF GOALS

As discussed at the start of this book, there is a clear task and societal goal for the hospital. However (Etzioni, 1964, p. 2), "The organization instead of being society's obedient servant, sometimes becomes its master." The goal which is the source of the hospital's legitimacy is the care and treatment of patients. However, during the time of this study the measure basic to allocation of funds was the average daily patient load, ADPL, and not the rate of recuperation or the size of the population served. A change to the size of population served might have featured results such as those reported by Moore *et al.* (1962) and Wilson *et al.* (1964) who found that approximately half the people usually considered appropriate for hospitalization can be effectively dealt with as outpatients. A change to a measure of recuperation as basic for allocation might have featured a report such as that by Bockoven (1963, p. vi) that Worcester State hospital was able to reduce its resident population by 40% while nearly doubling the number of people served (treated). This could not occur in the VA. A reduction in bed occupants (average daily patient load) (ADPL) would have meant a failure to fulfill mission and a concomitant reduction in basic allocation of funds. This situation is described by Kennard (1957, p. 43):

> At one medical staff meeting, the Chief of Professional Services announced that the hospital had been operating 100 or so beds under the average daily patient load necessary to maintain funds for the following year at the proper level. Within a month at a subsequent meeting, he announced that we would have to be more circumspect about admitting patients because we were by that time over the average daily patient load which was required.

There were strong pressures to keep the number of patients in the hospital up to a certain level; the hospital director had to do this to protect his employees. *The emphasis at the very root of funding was custodial treatment, for the measure was patients in beds, rather than patients in the community.* Because the basic allocation of funds is for a given number of patients per day, there are times when the hospital doors are wide open and patients are encouraged to enter so that the ADPL will be increased. Conversely, because additional funds are given only for food, when the number of patients grows greater than the established ADPL, entry into the hospital is made more difficult and intensive efforts are made to discharge patients currently hospitalized. It is impossible to say whether the ensuing dramatic increase in the discharge rate is due to the turning of staff effort from admission work-ups to discharge procedures or the administrative pressure and reinforcement for the behavior of discharging patients. Kennard provides an illustration of how an administrative change may affect treatment. In a hospital in which few patients had ground privileges, 254 beds previously reserved for tuberculosis patients were made available for psychiatric patients. To quote Kennard (1957, p. 43):

> Within two months of the time that 254 beds on the Convalescent Service became available, 254 patients from locked wards were found and transferred to this service. It is difficult to escape the conclusion that availability of this space in the hospital, rather than any radical change in the behavior of these patients, was the primary factor responsible for the granting of full ground-privileges.

*When ADPL is either too high or too low, the "needs of the organization" imposed by the method of funding appears to take precedence over either the staff's professional standards or the patient's needs. The clearest indication of this pressure in the data of the present study is the significant favorable correlation between new applications per bed and both measures of effectiveness.* The impact of the method of funding on an organization is not unique to VA hospitals and has been described by Clark (1961) for adult education in California. Briefly, funds were based on enrollment, and this in turn led to many "frill" courses which would attract students. This being the case, the professional status of adult education teachers decreased. The short-run need for clientele set by the enrollment economy was at variance with the long-run need for educational respectability as the basis for legitimacy.

## SITE OF FUNDING AND DISPLACEMENT OF GOALS

An organization displaces its goal when it "substitutes for its legitimate goal some other goal for which it was not created, for which resources were not allocated to it, and which it is not known to serve" (Etzioni, 1964, p. 10). One effect of the distance between the hospital and the central site of funding was the behavior likely to be reinforced. In the immediately foregoing section we suggested that the very basis of the allocation of funds was oriented to custody rather than treatment. Given this circumstance, what behavior would be so visible that the administrators and supervisors could observe and provide reinforcement? In the passage from Worthy (1950, p.176) previously quoted, we may find a clue: ". . . the individual supervisor or manager is under compulsion to operate in such a manner as to make a good showing in terms of the particular set of controls to which he is subject. . . ." In a similar fashion, Blau and Scott (1962, p. 185) remark; "It appears that management's primary significance is no longer as the apex of the authority pyramid; rather its central function is to design, in collaboration with a staff of experts, appropriate impersonal mechanisms of control." Foremost among these are records of work (Blau and Scott, 1962, pp. 178–80). But management must have a clear understanding of what it wishes to accomplish by these reports lest the reports become very selective of information, tend to minimize problems, emphasize success, and eventually mislead rather than inform. In short, attention is a generalized reinforcer and when given to a particular area of action by management, action will increase in that area. The point is elegantly made by Henry (1964, p. 32) in a study of nurses:

> "When you go off duty, they don't know whether you have spent time with the patients, but they do know whether you have written in the chart." This raises the important ancillary problem of the *hidden deficit*, which may be stated as follows: when a subordinate worker has a choice of tasks of unequal visibility, he will tend to perform the task of greater visibility and neglect the task of lower visibility—visibility referring, of course, not to what the worker sees, but rather to what his supervisor can see.

A first visible and reinforced behavior dealt with being "cost conscious." Stotland and Kobler (1965) and Cumming and Cumming (1956) have shown how control of funds, particularly when they are scarce, leaves the locus of power with the person, usually not one trained in the treatment of patients, who is most involved with funds. At a hospital level, the laboratory and administrative cost for a psychiatric admission can parallel the expense for a general medical admission, yet the funds allocated per psychiatric patient are approximately half of those for each general medical patient. A foundation of continued treatment, back ward patients, receiving a minimum of professional attention can help balance the books. Further, on a ward level each discharged patient has to be replaced by another patient.

Both admission and discharge mean a psychiatric "workup." Especially where the ideal is a stabilized ward in which a minimum amount of work (and treatment personnel) can deal satisfactorily with the largest number of patients, treatment and discharge can become negative occurrences because they imply extra work.

Another matter which is visible in reports stems from conceptions of necessary functions. These concepts are similar to values as defined by Parsons (1951, p. 12): "An element of a shared symbolic system which serves as a criterion or standard for selection among the alternatives of orientation which are intrinsically open in a situation may be called a value." Other things being equal, government personnel seem to value the image of private industry and think that the report of management conferences, staff development, and inservice training programs are particularly desirable. However, to be useful, inservice training must be germane to the situation and actually applied. To the extent that the line function in a psychiatric hospital is professional, it is possible to wonder how much can be accomplished by administrative inservice training programs. One example in my experience was a "Plain Letters" course in which two full days were spent learning how to write letters that were "short, simple, strong, and sincere." Secretaries who did not write letters to clients or other agencies were participants, as were physicians and scientists whose writing was a professional matter.

Two favored symbols at the time of this study were "communications" and "human relations." While genuine patient and staff interaction may be a major technique for avoiding the bureaucratic tendencies of the large public hospital, a technique without purpose may become a ritual.

Etzioni (1960) has written a careful review of the uncritical application of the industrial pattern of "human relations" and "communications" to psychiatric hospital settings. Discussing an instance reported by Caudill (1958) in which the wishes of the nurses and patients were in conflict, Etzioni writes:

> . . . it seems that the training of the hospital head prevented him from seeing the significance of these simple facts. Moreover, it seems that no additional communication about these factors could change them. . . . Like so many conflicts of interest, this one was solved by *bargaining* and *compromise* and not by a sheer increase in communication.

Neither the patient nor staff meetings served as a genuine source of communication. Rather, to quote Etzioni (1960):

> A detailed analysis of the material supplied by Caudill shows that these conferences are either manipulative or blocks to communication, and serve as a source of anxiety rather than as a positive influence. Stanton and Schwartz reach a similar conclusion in their discussion of staff conferences in another mental hospital. They state: "Conferences and discussions were regarded *as a means of rationalizing hospital interference*, and as discussions which might interfere with clear personal insight into the problem" [italics added by Etzioni].

The ideology of communications and human relations may be avidly embraced in psychiatric hospitals because the psychological, social work, and psychoanalytic background of the professional employees emphasizes far more than industry the importance of interpersonal relations. Given a dynamic, psychiatric background, the conviction may develop, through analogy, that talking about problems is "good," because talk leads to insight and insight to cure of otherwise hidden conflicts. Wallace and Rashkis (1959) present data questioning this view and Etzioni (1960) shows how it may be unrealistic and oversimplified. Holmes (1964, p. 206), who deals at length with the residential treatment of adolescents, writes: "Knowing what caused his need does not repair the deficiency any more than understanding the pathophysiology of itching diminishes the need to scratch." Even if insight is attained, there remains the problem of implementation.

Concurrent with a belief in communications, there may be an uncritical acceptance that the happiness of the worker is not only valuable in itself but a necessary condition for the effective performance of duties. The nature of the hospital situation and the professions of the people involved can heighten this belief. Walker (1961) in his extensive survey of civil service workers found the relation between efficiency and morale interesting only because it was so low. The strongest summary statement on the subject comes from Brayfield and Crockett (1955, p. 421) in a painstaking review article:

> We have arrived at two conclusions: first, that satisfaction with one's position in a network of relationships need not imply strong motivation to an outstanding performance within that system, and, second, that productivity may be only peripherally related to many of the goals toward which the industrial worker is striving. . . . Certain implications seem logical from the foregoing sections of this report. Foremost among these implications is the conclusion that it is time to question the strategic and ethical merits of selling to industrial concerns an assumed relationship between employee attitudes and employee performance. In the absence of more convincing evidence than is now at hand with regard to the beneficial effects on job performance of high morale, we are led to the conclusion that we might better forego publicizing these alleged effects.

A final verbal icon which may be maintained by its effectiveness in being accepted as a legitimate value is the phrase "for the good of the organization." As Allport (1933) points out, the referent in such a phrase is difficult to determine. One may ask, "for the good of the patients?" "for the good of the taxpaying public?" "for the good of the employees?" "for the preservation of the physical plant?" and draw negative answers to all of these questions. The "good of the service" or the "good of the organization" usually has little reference to anything save the good of the person who utters this phrase to cover an action he would be hard put to justify otherwise. There may even be a Gresham's law of information in which data are withheld, for "the timing is inauspicious." Inferior and ungermane material which would be obsolete if adequate material were circulated, may be reported in the administrative channels. Incomplete data may have to precede adequate information, lest the former be never reported and the particular sub-organization made to look bad. This situation may be rationalized by the person responsible for directing the sub-organization as for the good of the larger organization which needs a group such as his.

## AUTHORITY AND DISPLACEMENT OF GOALS

In this section we will touch on the system of authority found in psychiatric hospitals. In the second chapter of this book, Worthy (1950, p. 176) was quoted to the effect that problems may become particularly acute when two closely related functions report up two different systems of standards and controls. Later in this section we shall cite Etzioni (1964, p. 27) on the same matter. We will start this section, however, with two descriptions of the situation in psychiatric hospitals. A first quotation is from Greenblatt *et al.* (1955, pp. 269–70):

> In many such instances, conflicting spheres of responsibility and interest, which in themselves sustained older ingroup tensions, necessitated requests and explanations going through long and often parallel lines of communication if problems were to be settled. One line of communication went from the ward via the doctor to the physician who was chief of that particular service, and from him to the chief of professional services; another went via the head nurse, through the supervising nurse to the chief nurse, and thence to the chief of professional services. Different lines of communication were required when another department was involved, such as rehabilitation with its many specialized services. When information about a particular problem upon which decisions had to be based finally

reached the chief of professional services, it was so modified through being passed on by several persons that the nature of the original problem was frequently altered. Thus, the eventual decision was often inappropriate to the actual situation, or the situation had changed enough during the time consumed that opportunity and initiative were lost on the ward.

Kahne (1959) makes a similar point:

> In mental hospitals, the ward is the primary unit of social organization, yet in most hospitals the functional and scalar organization seriously interferes with the cohesion in its daily life. Physicians, nurses, aides, housekeepers, and other service personnel such as kitchen help all have independent chains of communication and command. As a result they often find themselves in institutionally induced conflict between responsibility to their own functional group and identification with the ward. The chronic necessity to serve multiple superiors whose aims are frequently tangential to each other tends to reduce their activity to a relatively indifferent, mechanical level. . . .

The situation on the ward may become one in which the psychiatrist has no choice over the selection of his nurse, psychologist, social worker, or secretary. He cannot hire, fire, or discipline them. He has no direct power in seeing that his orders are carried out. If he has a complaint, he either has to pursue the matter informally or complain to his supervisor who may then discuss the matter with the chief of the relevant service who in turn may discuss the matter with the employee. The chief of a professional service can transfer the employee to another ward, but he makes his decision without knowledge of the particular work situation other than reports from those involved. The person with responsibility on the ward for patients is in a very poor strategic situation: he is dependent upon the chief of the professional service to which the employee belongs. The chief of that service has a vested interest, the morale of his employees, and is not unlikely to side with the worker against a member of a different profession.

The absence of frequent, rapidly applied differential rewards may lead to a need to rely on interpersonal relationships and persuasion in order to get things accomplished (Bennis *et al.*, 1958). The psychiatrist may feel pressure to be a "nice guy" and run his ward in a manner approved of by other services. If he does not fulfill this requirement, heads of other services may assign him their least competent workers. The psychiatrist may complain and be assigned another incompetent. After two or three changes, the burden of proof comes to rest on the psychiatrist for he has been shown to be a person who can not get along with other people. In the world of mental health professionals, not to be able to get along with other people, "to have difficulties in interpersonal relations," is extremely damaging. In part it equates the person with mental patients, in part it permits anything the person says to be discounted *ad hominum.* The strength of such argument is noted by Stanton and Schwartz (1954, p. 205) who write that "... modern psychiatrists and psychologists make up one of the few groups in history where *ad hominum* argument may be treated with greater prestige than an argument confined to the subject matter of the discussion." The result is that the psychiatrist may feel forced to curry favor with the chiefs of other professional services. He has to fit in with the social customs of getting along, or he may be left with responsibility for patients without an effective staff. In the hands of some ancillary service chiefs shaping psychiatrists can become an art. For example, if there is less than one worker available per ward, the chief of an ancillary profession can assign two wards to a worker and leave to the worker's "discretion" the division of his time between the two wards. Failure to produce on a given ward can be excused by the assignment to another. Another technique, one cited by Merton (1940), is to withhold vital information for which an official is responsible, and then when he complains, to flood him with all incoming documents including trivia that he must sort through to find material for which he is responsible. A third common technique is delay, a procedure well described by Dimock (1952, p. 404). If these pressures exist for psychiatrists, the reader may consider the pressures on the non-medical staff. Rushing (1964) presents pictures of the difficulties of social workers, nurses, psychologists, and a recreational specialist at a highly staffed teaching hospital.

There are two points to emphasize: the first is that there is pressure on the topmost profession to conform to the mode of getting along. The second is the effect of organizational structure. To quote again from Etzioni (1964, p. 27), "Providing for any two employees and for any two organizational units, one point of authority to which both are subordinate and at which conflicts can be settled is viewed as essential to organizational efficiency." Further, noting the work of Simon, Smithburg, and Thompson (1954), Etzioni (1964, p. 27) points out that conflict should be resolved at as low a level in the hierarchy as possible:

> Low-level settlement reduces the work load of the most burdened and most "expensive" higher-level executives. It permits rapid settlement of disagreements since the lines of communication are shorter, and it permits the executive who

must serve as judge or arbiter to have a relatively full command of the facts and to be able to draw on his personal knowledge of the conflicting parties.

We touched on the difficulty in dealing with incompetent personnel. Walker (1961) studied British workers in two private companies and two Civil Service Ministries. There were 624 private office workers and 1067 civil servants who responded to the question of how incompetent people were dealt with. In both the Civil Service and private concerns, roughly one in five respondents reported that incompetents were allowed to stay where they were. The most frequent response (43.2%) by private concern employees was that incompetents are given one more chance and then gotten rid of. Only 15.8% of civil servants gave this response. The most frequent answer (63.5%) for the civil service employees was that incompetents are put where they will do the least harm, a response given by only 33.1% of private office workers. An interesting additional piece of information is that as the status of the job increased, the number of civil servants who reported that incompetents are put where they will do the least harm also increased. Clerical workers gave this response in 55.9% of the cases while administrative and professional personnel used it 73.6% and 72.3% of the time respectively. Davis (1948) offers corroboration from a different bureaucratic setting, the Navy. He described the tendency to avoid responsibility and do the least possible amount of work. Davis notes that business corporations counteract tendencies to avoid responsibility and work by making rewards depend heavily on individual initiative. "These incentives and sanctions are less available to the Navy, where seniority is primary and competition often operates negatively. Officer personnel are seldom dismissed, and then usually for offences against discipline rather than for incompetence." Henry (1954) notes that the organization can create interpersonal stresses and conflicts and therefore it is more parsimonious to investigate organizational structure prior to interpersonal relations:

Yet failure of a member to function adequately in an organization ought not to be too readily diagnosed as a symptom of some deep-going psychopathology—a point which may be particularly important to remember in an organization containing many persons skilled in psychiatric diagnosis. Rather, so it seems to me, in the presence of poorly functioning personnel, an administrator might ask himself *first* whether the poor functioning might not be due to some underlying defect in the organizational structure. It is not possible to put a group of even basically well-integrated persons into a poorly conceived organization and expect them to function without much stress.

## BUREAUCRACY AND DISPLACEMENT OF GOALS

In the introductory and data sections we indicated that large size was likely to be associated with negative effects. Dimock (1952, p. 398) writes: "There is likely to be a direct relationship between the size of an institution and its bureaucratic tendencies. The larger it becomes, the more pronounced is the tendency toward red tape; the smaller its size, the freer it is likely to be of inflexibilities."

Bureaucracy is a technique for organizing the efforts of many people toward a common goal. In theory, bureaucracy is purely rational, but in practice there are a number of undesirable effects as people accommodate to such a system. In this section we will discuss these effects as they may be manifested in large public psychiatric hospitals. While such hospitals are bureaucratic organizations, a point of equal importance is that they fail to meet the requirements defining situations for which bureaucracy is an appropriate way to organize the efforts of people. In short, psychiatric hospitals may suffer from most of the defects and obtain few of the benefits involved in bureaucratic organization.

In the following paragraphs, we will review some of the major theoretical characteristics of bureaucracy and discuss their relevance for psychiatric hospitals. In bureaucracy, there is, first, a continuous organization of official functions bound by rules. Rules save effort by obviating the need to derive a new solution for every problem and facilitate the standardization and equality of treatment of many cases. "These advantages are impossible if each client is treated as a unique case, as an individual" (Etzioni, 1964, p. 53). But we are dealing with a field of endeavor in which supposedly every case is unique. Official mental health ideology and bureaucratic concepts conflict on this point.

Second, in bureaucracy there is a systematic division of labor, rights, and power. The person must know his job, the limits of his job, and within the limits of his job, have the power to carry it out. In a psychiatric hospital the work of a professional person can be negated by another professional. For example, the importance of how a medicine is given has been noted in drug research and in the placebo effect. The nurse can be enthusiastic or apathetic. The aide can make fun of an activity to which he directs patients. The psychiatrist can deny a pass or privilege which the social worker or psychologist thinks would be therapeutic. The members of different professions may frequently consider each other as laymen when dealing with an area each considers within his specialty. To the extent that there is a great deal of overlap in the professional specialties treating psychiatric patients, a systematic division of labor, rights and power does not exist. Perrow (1965) goes further when he suggests that since a technology for treating psychiatric patients does not exist, a rational division of labor and authority cannot exist.

A third element of bureaucracy is that there is an organizational hierarchy in which each lower office is under supervisory control of the next higher so that no position is left uncontrolled, and in which no order avoids systematic checking and reinforcing. We have discussed how in the hospitals studied the members of one profession were supervised not by ward personnel but by members of their own profession. This extended to secretaries who did not work for their on-the-job supervisors (psychiatrists) but for the Registrar. Again, a ward psychiatrist had no direct power over the typing pool, the clothing room, the pharmacist, etc.

Fourth, the rules for conduct of an office are technical and their application is rational and by a person qualified on the basis of technical training. The root of the authority of the bureaucrat is presumably his knowledge and his training. We will note elsewhere that the most skilled persons, psychiatrists, psychologists, and social workers are, in these hospitals "line" rather than "staff." In a different manner we may draw on Etzioni (1964, p. 12) to illustrate the nonrational pressures on technical skill:

> For example, a welfare worker may fear the risks of making a decision on his own; he plays it safe by observing minutely the organization's rules and policies with the result that more important treatment considerations are underplayed. This is illustrated, for example, when a social worker in violation of his own judgment as to what would be most beneficial for the clients, recommends that a mentally disturbed child remain with his family, because the agency has a policy of not breaking up family units, even though the child's presence at home may disrupt the adjustment of the other children in the family. Instead of making procedures means to the organization's goal, he makes them ends in themselves. The policy becomes the prevailing criterion for decision, and the worker bends the clients' needs to fit the policy. Adherence to the organization's policy has become the organizational goal of the bureaucrat.

There is an additional pressure involved. In a professional group colleagues are the source of discipline while in bureaucracy the locus of discipline is the hierarchy of authority (Blau and Scott, 1962, p. 63). Additional professional training such as graduate work is likely to lead to a "cosmopolitan" orientation in which the person's reference group is located outside the organization (Blau and Scott, 1962, pp. 65–71, especially tables 1–3). Professional competence may therefore not only lead to conflict in applying rules to specific cases, it may lead to disloyalty and the difficulties described by Thompson (1963) in a subsequent section of this chapter.

A fifth aspect of bureaucracy is that administrative acts, decisions, and rules are formulated and recorded in writing. This is necessary to maintain a systematic interpretation of norms and enforcement of rules that cannot be maintained through oral communication. This practice also provides a continuity of history and acts beyond any individual servant. The mass of paper and rules is a very real part of life in the psychiatric hospital. Belknap (1956, p. 67) writes, "When the day to day role of the hospital physician is studied over a sufficient period of time, it becomes evident that as much as 60 per cent of his activity is usually devoted to work of an administrative nature." At times the production of paper becomes an end in itself, because paper, unlike interaction with patients, endures and is visible as "work accomplished" (Sharp, 1952; Gouldner, 1952; Henry, 1964).

An illustration of this aspect of hospital life and the close supervision (Blau and Scott (1962, p. 177): "An intensive downward flow of demands constitutes close supervision, a practice which tends to impede effective performance . . .") which may occur in bureaucratic organizations, is a hospital memorandum (5024/136 dated August 31, 1964) on the subject of "Psychiatric Patients' Handkerchiefs." The reader should be advised that "DM&S" refers to the Washington, D.C. Central Office of the organization: "Recently, DM&S Circular 10–64–82, April 1, 1964, discontinued the gratuitous issue to psychiatric patients of many incidental items, including handkerchiefs. . . . The use of handkerchiefs has, as expected, decreased markedly since the receipt of the above circular."

There are two conditions for effective bureaucracy which are met by public psychiatric hospitals. The members of the administrative staff should be completely separated from ownership of the means of production or administration. Further, in order to enhance organizational freedom, the organization should be free from outside control and the positions free from monopolization by any incumbent.

In a major contribution, Merton (1940) delineated the effects of working within a bureaucratic setting. Merton's analysis starts with the concept of a formal, rational organization in which action takes place through clearly defined rules "which preclude the necessity for issuance of specific instructions for each specific case. The generality of rules requires the constant use of *categorization*, whereby individual problems and cases are classified on the basis of designated criteria and are treated accordingly." However, when situations change it is easier to try to categorize them as appropriate to the old rules rather than to devise new ones. The very success of prior training may lead to inappropriate behaviour in new situations.

This emphasis on rules may lead to rules that were originally conceived as means being transformed into ends in themselves. This is another illustration of displacement. Merton argues that the person placed in a situation in which there is an over-concern with rules is likely to become timid, conservative, and formalistic. Especially in dealing with the public, the bureaucrat is likely to become impersonal as he resorts to categorization and precedent and avoids the "special features" which are important to the client but a hindrance to a stereotyped response. There is a tendency for such behavior to be seen by the client as arrogance. There is also the tendency, noted by Merton, for fellow workers who have identified themselves with the legitimacy of these rules to be antagonistic toward anyone who does not conform to them.

This major article by Merton (1940) (reprinted in Etzioni, 1961; Kluckhohn & Murray, 1950; Merton *et al.*, 1952) indicates how the organization of the environment channels behavior and tends to teach a person his proper role.

While I agree with Merton's observation of the impersonality and seeming arrogance in the behavior of employees *vis-à-vis* clients, I would like to add that there may be, beyond organizational structure, an additional explanation for this behavior. Once a person has been reprimanded by his supervisor for becoming "over-involved" with his client, he will do a lot to avoid the situation in the future. New employees are in for experiences not dissimilar to those of patients. They are taught not to cause trouble and exceptions to rules (the exigencies of individual cases or novel situations) are trouble. The trainee can, and is, asked why he got involved. The burden of proof is on him to show that it was not some blind spot or imperfection on his part. Another way of saying this is to note that the trainee must show that he acted correctly or professionally *when in fact he did something which his supervisor would not have done.* An employee learns to adopt a cold non-reinforcing attitude towards clients so that they will not continue to talk and produce information that puts him in conflict. Krasner (1958) describes the extent to which conversation can be controlled through verbal conditioning, and Davis (1948) provides an illustration of how far an avoidance of supervisory displeasure may lead to deviation from the purposes of the organization. Davis notes that heavy bomber crews on anti-submarine patrols usually made several errors in the course of an attack and would be sharply criticized by their superiors. This led to the practice of flying "quiet patrols" in which the letter of the flight instructions were obeyed legalistically. If a suspicious object appeared a few miles to one side or the other of their charted course, the pilot's path lay straight ahead.

There are situations conducive to deviation from impersonal, rational adherence to rules. Francis and Stone (1956) investigated whether or not bureaucracy implied a dominant emphasis on impersonality and procedure. Their major finding was that there were conflicting patterns rather than one dominant pattern. While they noted that rule-following and service to clients sometimes conflicted, there was an orientation of service and an orientation which stemmed from a moral attitude about the dispensation of money (in an Employment Security Office). Agency procedures were considered a means to the end of aiding deserving clients or a means of sustaining a decision to disallow a claim. Analysing the completion of a large number of forms, Francis and Stone found several pragmatic factors dictated deviations from set rules. These deviations aided in achieving a high percentage of job placements. Francis and Stone (1956, p. 129) note that:

> The factors causing deviation from manual rules were: (1) pressure for high productivity, i.e., serving many clients per hour; (2) special skills involved in job placement which negated at certain points the underlying theory on which the forms were developed; (3) rush orders that forced abandonment of procedures; (4) cultural attitudes that caused differential treatment of Negro and white clients.

There was a definite emphasis on productivity which was consciously and overtly directed toward a justification of the agency's budget. If they could not provide objective indices of work, they feared their budget would be cut by Congress.

A second aspect which may account for deviation from an

impersonal and procedure orientation is that the people who were studied had direct contact with clients. Francis and Stone hypothesize that (1956, pp. 160–1):

> In contrast to the interviewers, let us consider those people who make up staff and middle management groups. These people do not directly supervise interviewers or deal with clients, but rather have as their main task the administration of the rules and procedures or the development of new rules and procedures. If the very content of the task consists largely in the administration of rules, then it may be that such people tend to conceive of the rules as ends in themselves in order to successfully carry out their tasks. If this is true, and if the professional principle does not operate as strongly for these people, then one might expect that such functionaries would be closely attached to the bureaucratic mode of operation.

Francis and Stone cite the work of Robert Dubin (1951, p. 155) and Gardner and Moore (1952, pp. 55–56) to substantiate this point. The latter authors are quoted as follows:

> Department chiefs generally identify themselves with management much more than foremen do. They seem to be much more "management minded"; they show much more interest in costs and efficiency; and they accept the rules more completely. This may be the result of their separation from the work itself, plus their increased participation in planning, coordination, and contacts up the line.

Data which supplement and extend the work of Francis and Stone (1956) are presented by Blau (1963). When records of accomplished work were initiated in a public employment agency, placement operations improved considerably. Despite a decrease in job openings, number of placements increased (Blau, 1963, table 1, p. 39). Of great interest were the side-effects associated with the change. On the one hand job finding, which was tabulated, increased in emphasis over vocational counseling. On the other hand, while (Blau, 1963, p. 94) "Negroes were discriminated against at the reception desk, where operations were not evaluated on the basis of statistical records," the greater likelihood of Negroes following through on job placement led to an increase of their placement. To quote Blau (1963, p. 94): "If objectives of overriding importance can be made to govern organized activities, discrimination will be eliminated regardless of the presence of prejudice."

A study which makes explicit the distinction between task orientation and organizational orientation is by Udy (1959). Using 150 formal organizations in 150 non-industrial societies, Udy found that three "bureaucratic" variables (A, hierarchical authority structure; B, specialized administrative staff; and C, rewards differentiated according to office) were all positively and significantly associated with each other. He found that four rational variables (D, limited organizational objectives such as production of goods; E, a performance emphasis; F, segmental participation based on mutual limited agreement; and G, compensatory rewards to lower authority members based on participation) were all positively associated with each other, five of the six possible associations being statistically significant. Finally, nine of the 12 associations between rational and bureaucratic characteristics were negatively associated with each other, and the only significant associations were between *presence* of B (specialized administrative staff) and *absence* of D, F and G defined above.

A series of studies which indicate deviation in practice from the ideal bureaucratic pattern focuses on a Navy setting (Turner, 1947; Davis, 1948; Page, 1946). In line with the observation that contact with production is associated with greater flexibility in application of rules, it is worth noting that the closer the military situation comes to active combat, the less formal and bureaucratic it becomes. Turner's article describes a situation very similar to the one in the psychiatric hospital *between employees.*

The basic element in the situation described by Turner (1947) is that there are pressures applied by a number of informal structures not envisaged in the formal pattern. The disbursing officer handles matters (pay) of immediate importance to his clients and errors or delays are quickly noticed and protested. There can be conflict between immediate demands (including those of his superiors) and the regulations. There must be some *modus vivendi* established between written rules and immediate verbal orders. First there are *friendship patterns.* "As a human being the disbursing officer wants to help his friends, and the penalty for brusque disposal of such requests is social ostracism." Another pattern is called *simulated friendship* in which through compliments and equality of treatment a senior officer strives to be defined as a person rather than as an applicant at a later date. Of particular interest is what Turner called an *exchange system.* Within the division of labor in a bureaucracy, each person has some sphere of duties where he can delay, make difficulties, or give an applicant a bare minimum or second best quality. To quote Turner, "The exchange structures extend so far that it is often difficult for a man to secure those services and equipment which are essential to his job unless he can promise some return . . . even some enlisted men in key positions, such as the mail clerk and carpenter's mates, are able to exercise influence over officers because of the services at their disposal." Resort to strictly formal procedure may impair the disbursing officer's potentially good position in the system of mutual benefits.

While professional workers such as psychologists, psychiatrists, and social workers may have greater prestige than administrative and engineering employees, these employees, because they can delay services that are immediate and personal, are far from powerless. This situation generates pressure for conformity in a horizontal manner that complements the vertical pressures which will be described in the following section on supervision. A person who acquires the reputation for being "pushy" or a "sorehead" may experience aversive consequences as long lasting as they are unforeseeable.

Turner makes this point when he notes, "The exchange system incorporates its own code of behavior. The individual who puts legal technicality ahead of reciprocity is reprehensible, is spoken of with almost moral indignation. The system is supposed to operate in leisurely fashion, maintaining the appearance that the goods acquired are secondary to the friendships involved." What is perhaps most important here is that a "personal" approach takes the place of an impersonal one. The rules are present as a threat, as a method by which red tape can be brought into play to delay any needed action. Given this background, two generalizations offered by Turner hold true for the psychiatric hospital. First, these informal systems "operate not only to grant favors to some but to withhold fair consideration from others." To quote Turner, "Because of the time consumed in extra-routine treatment of persons on the 'in,' others get summary treatment." The efficiency of the organization is reduced by the realities of living within it. Loopholes in regulations can become tools by means of which a bureaucrat elevates his own status and increases his own bargaining power. A second point made by Turner is that "Prompt careful attention to the business of a client is often defined as a favor."

The presence of negotiation and convenient application of rules was described by Turner. Strauss *et al.* (1963, pp. 151–6) illustrate this situation in the psychiatric hospital setting:

> In Michael Reese, as unquestionably in most sizable establishments, hardly anyone knows all the extant rules, much less exactly what situations they apply to, for whom, and with what sanctions. If this would not otherwise be so in our hospital, it would be true anyway because of the considerable turnover of nursing staff. Also noticeable—to us as observers—was that some rules once promulgated

would fall into disuse, or would periodically receive administrative reiteration after the staff had either ignored those rules or forgotten them. . . .

As in other establishments, personnel called upon certain rules to obtain what they themselves wished. Thus the nurses frequently acted as virtual guardians of the hospital against some demands of certain attending physicians. . . . As elsewhere, too, all categories of personnel are adept at breaking the rules when it suits convenience or when warrantable exigencies arise. Stretching the rules is only a further variant of this tactic, which itself is less attributable to human nature than to an honest desire to get things accomplished as they ought, properly, to get done. Of course, respective parties must strike bargains for these actions to occur.

Strauss *et al.* note that numerous examples are provided by Dalton (1959, especially pp. 104–7).

However, yet another ground of negotiation needs emphasizing: namely, that in this hospital, as doubtless elsewhere, the patient as an "individual case" is taken as a virtual article of faith. By this we mean that the element of medical uncertainty is so great, and each patient is taken as—in some sense—so unique, that action around and about him must be tailor-made, must be suited to his precise therapeutic requirements. This kind of assumption abets what would occur anyhow: that only a minimum of rules can be laid down for running a hospital, since a huge area of contingency necessarily lies outside those rules. The rules can provide guidance and command for only a small amount of the total concerted action that must go on around the patient. It follows, as already noted, that where action is not ruled it must be agreed upon.

Negotiation may well be a necessary outgrowth of the related variables of size and complexity. Gardner and Moore (1952, p. 80, quoted in Francis and Stone, 1956, p. 159) give a general statement of this problem:

Every job, every department in an organization, by the very nature of the functions which it is called upon to perform, develops a certain set of demands on other jobs and departments in the organization. Out of these demands grow many of the stresses and strains and the potential for conflict which are characteristic of industrial organizations. . . . As the division of labor becomes more complex, it can be seen that the demands become correspondingly proliferated and intense. . . . It is apparent from this that the potential for conflict among employees increases with the complexity of its technology and its size.

Kahne (1959) applies these points directly to the mental hospital situation:

The more highly specialized the departments, the more difficult it is to secure a consensus; principles acceptable to everyone will necessarily be general formulations which can encompass their biases. Furthermore, hierarchy makes the legitimacy of an opinion mostly a reflection of status, and since control over formal communication rests inevitably with higher echelons, "official" patient needs usually represent the opinions of upper-level personnel. Because task fragmentation in mental hospitals means that upper-level personnel are most distant from the patient, their formulations about patient needs are invariably based upon the needs of patients in general.

Kahne (1959) also reports a circumstance which is similar to Turner's discussion of the naval situation: "At the ward level, routines occupy the center of the stage, and, curiously enough, response to individual needs is regarded as *special treatment.*"

A final quotation, one from Dunham and Weinberg (1960, p. 64), may serve to summarize the total effect of bureaucratic pressures within the psychiatric hospital:

> While lip-service is always given to new ideas, constant obstacles are thrown in the path of any person in any one of these groups who may want to get something done. For getting something done quickly, accurately, and efficiently is perhaps the most basic sin anyone can commit within the hospital society. This is particularly true because the desire of any person to introduce something new is likely to be disturbing to someone else who has a vested interest in some aspect of hospital life.

## SUPERVISORY BEHAVIOR AND DISPLACEMENT

The psychiatric hospital shares problems common to all bureaucratic modern organizations. These problems are heightened by (a) the separation between the employee and either taxpayer or patient, (b) the personal rather than material focus of psychiatric treatment, and (c) the lines of authority which are drawn along professional rather than functional distinctions. In this situation, the focus of immediate supervision is displaced from patient care to satisfying the person on the next step of the hierarchy. These points have been discussed by Victor Thompson in his *Modern Organization* (1963).

Thompson starts his analysis with the attempt by modern bureaucracy to fit professional and technical specialization into a traditional hierarchical framework. Technicians have the ability to make decisions which persons with hierarchical status have the right to make. "In short, *the most symptomatic characteristic of modern bureaucracy is the growing imbalance between ability and authority*" (Thompson, 1963, p. 5). Further, "Authority is centralized, but ability is inherently decentralized because it comes from practice rather than from definition. Whereas the boss retains his full *rights* to make all decisions, he has less and less *ability* to do so because of the advance of science and technology" (Thompson, 1963, p. 47).

Turning to the focus of the present section, reinforcement of employee behavior in the institutional setting, we can follow

Thompson (1963, p. 61) when he makes a number of points introduced earlier in this chapter:

> Although there are many promotional arrangements, nearly all depend heavily and ultimately on the kind word from the "boss." . . . Hierarchical relations overemphasize the veto and under-emphasize approval of innovation. Since there is no appeal from the superior's decision, a veto usually ends the matter. However, an approval will often have to go to a next higher level where it is again subject to a veto. A hierarchical system, therefore, always favors the status quo.

Thompson refers to Leavitt (1958, pp. 259–62), Moore (1951, p. 143), and Powell (1956, pp. 395–8) for further documentation of this point. Other matters are also touched on: specific standards of a public nature detract from the authority of the "boss"; the superior controls the official channels of communication and "appeal" is either an illegitimate procedure or one leading to a deterioration of relations with the boss whose decision is challenged; the burden of proof is on the employee rather than the boss.

As one moves up the hierarchy the standard of performance becomes more personal, vague, and covert, as does the performance of duties. Thompson (1963, pp. 67–8) notes the tendency for people to impute superior abilities to persons of higher status and call upon them to help solve all sorts of problems including those about which they have no knowledge whatsoever:

> In public affairs, this halo effect of status requires high-status persons to speak out on all sorts of matters from a position of almost complete ignorance. They are, therefore, forced to develop plausible-sounding jargons and propositions which come to constitute pseudo-technologies in terms of which many of our public problems must be publicly analyzed and discussed.

In the psychiatric hospital Kahne (1959) observed the use of jargon as a status enhancing activity. A related status producing activity is speech at staff meetings. Caudill (1958) noted that the higher the status of the person, the more frequently he spoke at staff meetings. Speaking in groups regardless of content, is positively associated with evaluation of having made a contribution (Hastorf, 1965). The upward-mobile staff member talks frequently in a manner valued by his superior.

Moore (1951, p. 143) and March and Simon (1958, p. 63) and notably Thompson (1963, pp. 72–3) have pointed out:

> . . . that there are few operational performance standards for hierarchical positions. Incumbents can never be sure "how well they are doing." Their activities have less and less of specialist content and become more and more purely hierarchical role playing. . . . As one goes up the hierarchy, therefore, he has less and

less value for other organizations. These two conditions—lack of operational performance standards and lack of opportunities in other organizations—make for great anxiety. This anxiety is most likely to express itself in a neurotic over-emphasis on pleasing the boss, which serves only to increase the boss's self-evaluation and therefore his demands for deference.

Given this background, Thompson (1963, p. 82) notes that "To realize his personal goals in the organization, the subordinate has to please the boss, whatever this requires. Technical competence is not enough." Further, Thompson (1963, p. 91) cites Whyte (1957, pp. 143 ff.) and notes ". . . the growing antipathy to idea men, to brilliance, that pervades our bureaucracies. The average person who will *get along* with others and *go along* with the system is preferred." The specialist finds that the greatest rewards are in non-technical work and therefore he must play the game.

"Thus 'brown-nosing,' hypocrisy, and 'false personalization' are endemic in modern bureaucracies" (Thompson, 1963, p. 94). The specialist must give up his particular skills if he wishes to be a "success" in hierarchical competition, and "A corollary of the hierarchical appropriation of success is the derogation of intellect, imagination, and skill so prevalent in modern bureaucracy" (Thompson, 1963, p. 97).

Reference can be made to Whyte (1957), Riesman, Glazer, and Denney (1950), Fromm (1941), and particularly the description of the marketing orientation (Fromm, 1947) in which man treats himself as a commodity to be validated by how well he can sell himself. The person to whom the employee sells himself is his supervisor. "The crucial questions are not merit and ability in the ordinary sense, but the compatability and loyalty of the newcomers from the standpoint of the existing management 'team.' 'Is he our kind?' " (Thompson, 1963, p. 98). Aside from rewarding those who do as they wish, hierarchical superiors by personalizing decisions function at a level in keeping with their limited technical ability. By operating at the level of individuals and personal problems, the need to seek overt standards, to question, and perhaps to revise the existing situation is avoided.

A variant of personalizing decisions is the therapy-oriented or psychiatric approach to supervision (Blau and Scott, 1962, pp. 188–91). Failure to conform to directives may be analyzed as an indication of unconscious resistance. The supervisor need not demonstrate that his judgment is superior in terms of professional or other objective standards, and may dismiss the worker's defense of himself as a "rationalization." Perhaps the most effective counter-maneuver to such supervision is for the employee to request psychological help from his supervisor. The supervisor can fulfill his role as a "good supervisor" by treating his employee therapeutically. He can then validate his own competence through gains made by his employee, i.e. job benefits which he himself manipulates.

Therapeutic supervision may be contrasted with the use of objective performance records (Blau and Scott, 1962, pp. 178–9, 248). Aside from exerting a direct influence on performance (e.g. our prior quotation from Blau, 1963, p. 94), Blau and Scott list the following effects of performance records: the supervisor no longer needed to check frequently on the work of subordinates, he could let records speak for themselves and not antagonize workers by telling them their work was poor, he could focus on accomplished results and permit subordinates greater discretion as to choice of procedures, he could assume the role of an adviser whose function was to help improve rather than judge employees' performance. Another desirable effect of the use of performance records is presented by Blau and Scott (1962, p. 179): "The freedom from close supervision and rigid operating rules that performance records make possible tends to enhance work satisfaction." This finding is in line with a more general concept provided by Blau and Scott (1962, p. 153): "Effective leadership requires not only refraining from closely checking on subordinates but it also requires making challenging demands to stimulate their interest and, indeed, their ability to perform well."

The assignment of a task rather than a procedure will be discussed in Chapter 11 in terms of "job enlargement" or "simple undifferentiated subordination." At this time, three issues need to be touched on. The first is that the larger the hospital or the longer the supervisory chain, the more likely the only feedback the superior obtains is behavior in conferences or hearsay reports. To get things done, illegal or unsanctioned procedures, which cannot be reported, may be used. This may be in the form of communication and negotiation out of channels or in the form of unreported treatment. To refer once more to Kahne (1959): "Lower-level personnel become more covert in activities which they regard as relevant, since their position in the hierarchy renders hazardous any sustained attempt to go counter to established authority." That is, personalized service, innovations, and individualized treatment may become risks rather than reinforced behavior.

The second issue is an important caution. The quotation which concludes the summary to this chapter was selected to indicate both the control exerted by performance records and the effect of poor selection, definition, or follow-up of such quantitative procedures. Performance records are means and not ends and their unsophisticated use is as open to criticism as the unspecific use of verbal symbols such as "human relations" and "the good of the organization."

The third and final issue is an attempt to describe what behavior is likely to be reinforced in the absence of overt standards and records. Thompson (1963) points out the increasing emphasis on skillfully acting the hierarchical role and the steady decline of the importance of competence. For example (Thompson, 1963, p. 142):

> The dramaturgical management of impressions about hierarchical positions and roles is no longer a sporadic affair depending upon the accidents of personality. It appears to be institutionally organized. That is to say, opportunities for hierarchical success in modern bureaucracy depend to a very large extent upon the ability and willingness to engage in impression management.

And again, (Thompson, 1963, p. 149):

> It is especially important in the selection process to determine the discretion of the person to be admitted to the team. He must have no black spots on his record; and a good record is most easily achieved by "going along with the gang," by avoiding risky innovations or ideas. He must not appear too intellectual, nor too technically skilled; and he must at least appear to place the good of the team above his profession.

Preparation and selection for administrative posts may have little relation to professional competence, but much with the ability to get along and be like the supervisor. Riesman, Glazer, and Denney (1950), Whyte (1957), and Etzioni (1964) are among the authors who have noted the spread of sociability beyond the work situation. The people selected for promotion parallel the supervisors who select them. The organizational and personal interests of administrative and treatment personnel may increasingly diverge.

One indication of such divergence is provided by informal association (see also Mishler and Tropp, 1956). Other than a shortage of seats or the peculiar geographical and organizational mobility of bachelors toward attractive females, groupings during lunch and coffee breaks in the canteen provided a rapid estimate of informal organization. Chiefs of professional services were likely to gravitate towards chiefs of administrative services rather than fellow professionals. It is difficult to say whether a particular type of person will move toward administrative activities or whether having become an administrator a person's views are likely to change.[1] In either case there is an effect on what is important in the work situation and what leisure time activities are of interest. Aside from differences in content, differences in epistemology may arise: the administrator may focus on what works in a particular organization or even with a particular superior. The professional person whose task involves clients or research may find himself more readily understood by a member of a different profession who works in the same situation than a member of his own profession who is hierarchically oriented. This situation is involved in the suggestion to be made in Chapter 11 that the powers of functional supervisors such as ward psychiatrists be increased.

A different aspect of displacement of goals in the supervisory process involves the behavior for which the supervisor is reinforced. Aside from pleasing his supervisor, there were, at the time of the present study, two bases for promotion in the government service. A first consideration was supervisory responsibility. In terms of career advancement, the classification system rewarded *increasing* the number of people doing a job rather than efficiency as measured by *decreasing* the number of people needed for a task. Parkinson's first law (1957) deals with both the background and the techniques used to fill the time available for work. Given the friendship patterns, the exchange system, and the absence of adherence to ostensible purposes (e.g. the first section of this chapter on the basis for funding), advancement through increases in personnel supervised played a major role in the positive correlations among all forms of expenditure (see the second section of Chapter 10).

A second avenue for advancement was through reclassification of

[1] Data presented by Lieberman (1956) dealing with rank-and-file factory workers who became shop stewards and foremen and who, in a later phase of the study, reverted to the rank-and-file role, would argue for the importance of the position. The material presented by Kelly and Goldberg (1959, especially table 18, p. 21) would argue for the importance of the type of person. Kelly and Goldberg analyzed personality measures obtained at the start of graduate training for groups of subjects who later specialized within clinical psychology as administrators, therapists, or academicians (teachers and research workers). Compared to therapists and academicians, people who later became administrators were characterized at the time of starting professional training as low childhood rebelliousness, low intra-psychic conflict, high conventionality, low curiosity, high interest in political and economic values, low creativity, and high vocational indecisiveness.

positions. Those matters which were "more professional" were "grade enhancing." The evaluation of what deserved a higher salary, however, was not made with any reference to effectiveness with patients. Forms of diagnosis and treatment which were inferential were more likely to be grade enhancing than more direct procedures. For example, the administration and evaluation of a standardized or objective test such as the Stanford–Binet was not as grade-enhancing as a more abstruse procedure such as the interpretation of the Rorschach. The very characteristics of a technology which a scientist might value such as the elimination of variance due to individuals were in many instances opposed to grade enhancement. In practice, what employees may see reinforced and learn to model (Bandura, 1965) are administration-oriented rather than treatment-oriented practices. Status in many regards may depend on *not* interacting with patients. Contact with clients is concentrated at the lower levels of the organization, and, to quote Etzioni (1964, p. 100), ". . . those who are successful in their relations with clients find it more difficult to attain promotion than those who prepare themselves for the next less-client-oriented stage by being more organization- than client-oriented."

To return to the concept with which we started this section, ". . . the most basic principle of administrative authority and the most basic principle of authority based on knowledge—or professional authority—not only are not identical but are quite incompatible" (Etzioni, 1964, p. 76). Knowledge is largely an individual property and something which the individual brings with him and maintains as an individual activity. Creativity cannot be ordered, coordinated, or otherwise bureaucratically administered. The experience of being consumed by a meaningful problem has in it elements of the exhilaration and agony of love, and, like love, makes a person a bit mad. Finally:

> Even the application of knowledge is basically an individual act, at least in the sense that the individual professional has the ultimate responsibility for his professional decision. . . . Only if immune from ordinary social pressures and free to innovate, to experiment, to take risks without the usual social repercussions of failure, can a professional carry out his work effectively. It is this highly individualized principle which is diametrically opposed to the very essence of the organizational principle of control and coordination by superiors—i.e., the principle of administrative authority. In other words, the ultimate justification for a professional act is that it is, to the best of the professional's knowledge, the right act. . . . The ultimate justification of an administrative act, however, is that it is in line with the organization's rules and regulations, and that it has

been approved—directly or by implication—by a superior rank." (Etzioni, 1964, pp. 76–77.)

## SUMMARY

In this chapter we have discussed the situation at the large public psychiatric hospital with a view towards sketching the background in which the empirical results were obtained. We discussed five sources of displacement. As was pointed out by our quotation from Henry (1954), rather than placing blame for seemingly irrational behavior on some sickness in the individual, we should look first at the situation to which he is adjusting. Berne (1964, p. 19) indicates both the general approach and this specific idea when he writes, "Experience has shown that it is more useful and enlightening to investigate social transactions from the point of view of the advantages gained than to treat them as defensive operations." Behaviors which are at variance with the purposes of the organization may well be more frequently reinforced than behaviors which provide the needed service intended by those who support the institution.

Organisms adjusting to a situation, whether they be schizophrenics or paid personnel will emit the behaviors for which they are positively reinforced. The following quotation is presented to illustrate the reasonableness of the behavior of employees. It is also presented to illustrate how the accomplishment of original purposes must be constantly kept in mind: neither related purposes nor dependence on the internal motives of employees are sufficient to insure attainment of the societally desirable goal. Finally, there is an optimistic implication to this entire chapter: if employee behavior is responsive to one environment, it should be responsive to environments designed to foster appropriate behavior.

Since factory output goals are either laid down in weight or quota by the planners a knitwear plant ordered to produce 80,000 caps and sweaters naturally produced only caps: they were smaller and thus cheaper and quicker to make. A factory commanded to make lamp-shades made them all orange, since sticking to one color kept the assembly line uncomplicated. . . . Taxi drivers were put on a bonus system based on mileage, and soon the Moscow suburbs were full of empty taxis barreling down the boulevards to fatten their bonuses. . . . The more tons of chandeliers the plant produced, the more the workers earned in bonuses. The chandeliers grew heavier and heavier, until they started pulling the ceilings down. They fulfilled the plan, admitted Khruschchev angrily, "but who needs this plan? To whom does it give light?" (*Time*, February 12, 1965, p. 24.)

## CHAPTER 10

# *Empirical Results and the Hospital Context*

CHAPTER 8 listed a number of empirical findings as foci for discussion and Chapter 9 presented material about the hospital setting. This chapter will bring together the material of the two previous chapters. After indicating strengths and weaknesses, suggestions for improvement, the topic of Chapter 11, will follow logically.

## SIZE

One of the two major hypotheses with which this work began was that small size was positively associated with effectiveness. The empirical findings supported this hypothesis but also refined it greatly. Small size was indeed significantly associated favorably with rapid release even after staffing had been held constant by partial correlation. With staffing held constant, small size also showed a trend ($r = .30$) to be correlated with a low percentage of patients with long hospitalization. A second finding was that size did not add to the multiple correlations for rapid release and long hospitalization obtained when other selected variables were used.

In our introductory chapters we cited authors such as Indik and Barker to the effect that active participation might be facilitated by small size. In Chapter 9 size was touched on in our discussion of bureaucracy. The tenor of that discussion is reflected by the following citation from Presthus (1962, p. 11): "The importance of size for our purposes is that large number of employees and large-scale operations result in a bureaucratic situation whose structural characteristics and psychological climate evoke certain patterns of individual accommodation." Further (Presthus, 1962, p. 42) "The sheer number of members prohibits communication; and the resulting ignorance and inertia encourage direction by the few." To the extent that there is an avoidance of risks (a) numerous people have veto powers, (b) bottlenecks develop, and (c) the decision-making process becomes highly diffused. In Presthus's words (1962, p. 53) "organized irresponsibility" follows.

With increasing size there is an increasing number of administrative steps and supervisory levels. The opportunity to hide on the part of both supervisors and employees is increased. Unrealistic decisions, which may create a good image on paper for others even further removed, are cultivated. With increasing size, the chance for informal communication is decreased and is replaced by memoranda. The emphasis is on generality rather than the specifics of a given case.

The greater impact of size on early release than on long hospitalization is, I think, associated with this last effect. Smaller size is likely to lead to more personal service that maximizes the capacities the patient has on admission. The decision for discharge is likely to be more rapid and the efforts of the staff directed to the patient's individual problems. As time progresses, the effects of institutionalization are such that we may hypothesize that greater and more specific therapeutic efforts are needed.

## *PER DIEM* EXPENSE AND STAFFING

The second major hypothesis with which this work started was that increased staffing was positively associated with effectiveness. As with size, the hypothesis was supported, but in such a manner as to specify and limit the area of impact. A higher number of treatment staff per patient was significantly correlated with a lower percentage of patients with long, continued hospitalizations, but in general not significantly with a higher rate of early release.

A second major finding involved consistent positive correlations among all forms of expenditure. An increase in available funds meant an increase for all areas of expenditure. There was a relative lack of specificity in the application of funds that was both surprising and appalling. The range of *per diem* expense in various areas is presented in Appendix 3 of this book. As an example, the range of cost per patient per day for the area of housekeeping was from \$.19 to \$.78. Considering that ten cents a day per patient at a 1500-bed hospital would have provided an additional psychiatrist *and* social worker, it is reasonable to ask why one hospital spent \$.78 for housekeeping when it might have spent only \$.60 and hired additional treatment personnel.

In terms of the discussions in the previous chapter, the answer to the present question lies in the basis of promotions and channels of authority. The separation of different areas of work (Engineering, Housekeeping, Psychology, Social Work, etc.) ran through the hospital to the Area Offices and into the Veterans Administration's Central Office in Washington. The exchange system, introduced by our reference to Turner, operated in dividing additional funds so that all services increased. A "good" admin'strator had an expanding service. While decisions were theoretically made at the Central Office, Area Office, and hospital Manager's Office, rigorous allocations in terms of work were, as the correlations indicate, not made. The powers of service chiefs who had been slighted to disrupt, delay, and generally retaliate were sufficient to insure everyone eventually obtaining a share of increased funds. This was something an administrator would work hard for because his administrative image and his personal salary were involved. Presthus (1962, p. 23) writes that "Conviviality, 'personality' and dependency became major career skills." Nowhere were such skills more necessary or in greater evidence than in the administrator's maneuvers to increase his part of the budget. On an immediate level, the chief whose service was not getting as much money as comparable services at other hospitals was not being an effective administrator.

In a section on "Sharing the Wealth" Moore (1964, p. 119) makes a similar observation:

> A major source of the competitive spirit in budget-making is that budgets have symbolic as well as "real" significance. Even if an increased budget carries no direct financial benefit to the manager . . . the increase is a sign of success, a reward for well-doing, a mark of approval. To ask for a repetition of the previous budget, to say nothing of less money, may raise questions concerning the man's ambitions and other attributes of managerial virtue.

On a day-to-day level, one of the first things an administrator may do is find an excuse. For example, if he had numerous employees who had worked for the government many years, he could argue that he had to spend money because (a) his employees had high within-grade salaries and (b) their seniority led to their being in a higher vacation bracket so that at any given time more of them were on annual leave. If the employer did not have this problem, he could excuse his expenditure on the basis of high turnover or the need to hire people to make up for the lack of experience of his employees.

## GENERAL ADMINISTRATION

There were a number of findings in terms of expenditure for general administration. The first finding was that as size increased, *per diem* expense for general administration decreased ($r = -.69$). This relationship between size and *per diem* expense for general administration was even greater ($r = -.75$) when total *per diem* was held constant. Larger size may therefore be said to be associated with lower administrative overhead per patient. However, it was found that expenditure in the area of general administration was positively associated with the percentage of early first significant releases. It appears that something of worth was accomplished by expenditure in this area. An analysis of the components of expenditure indicated that increased expenditure in the area of the Registrar was favorably associated with measures of effectiveness while expenditure in the area of Personnel tended to be unfavorably associated with measures of effectiveness (see the lower half of Table 14). With size and %-psychiatric held constant by double-partial correlation, and total *per diem* by use of a percentage, the percentage of the total *per diem* accounted for by the Registrar was significantly and favorably associated with both early release (.55) and long hospitalization (—.39). In the parallel analysis there was a trend for a high percentage of the total *per diem* spent by Personnel to be associated with a low percentage of early release (—.27) and, if anything, a higher percentage of patients with long hospitalization (.17).

We may use the Registrar and Personnel data to indicate the manner in which work in the area of general administration may help or hinder the treatment of patients. The Registrar provides clerical and transcription services to the wards; reviews qualitative and quantitative standards of medical records; is custodian for patient's effects; provides hospital communications, messengers, and employee and patient travel service; and has a clerical function for the admission, maintenance, and disposition of eligible patients including the determination of eligibility for benefits, initiation of patient's records, administration of commitments, guardianships, insurance, and statistical and management control reports. Personnel functions in five areas: *staffing and employment* which includes merit promotion program, orientation of new employees, interviewing of applicants, and the separated career employee program; *classification and wage administration* which includes reviews, surveys, desk audits, supervisory reviews, classification and wage administration training, and the production of organizational and functional charts; *processing and records section* which includes establishment and maintenance of employee records and files; *employee development section* which includes the development of recommendations to the training committee, coordination of all administrative and employee development and training, and supervision of clerical documentation of various employee awards actions; and *employee-management relations section* which includes the conduct of performance evaluations, the development of programs working with unions and employee associations, employee information programs, and employee health programs such as annual physical exam. The Registrar performs tasks necessary in the treatment of patients while Personnel seems to create work for itself by creating work for others. The evaluation and training of treatment staff is beyond the competence of any but members of the treatment professions (see Blau and Scott, 1962, p. 63).

## FOOD AND SHELTER

Although all *per diem* expenses were positively associated with each other, the amount of money spent on food and shelter (Table 10) tended to be negatively associated with early release. When variations in size, %-psychiatric, and total *per diem* were taken into account, the percentage of the *per diem* spent for food and shelter was significantly associated in an unfavorable direction with both early release and long hospitalization. It should be noted that the correlation between the percentage of the *per diem* spent on food and shelter and the total *per diem*, after size and %-psychiatric had been held constant, was random. This indicates that what was involved went beyond an artifact in which an increase in the percentage of expense for food and shelter meant a decrease in treatment personnel.

The percentage of *per diem* spent on food and shelter may well reflect the orientation and balance of power existing at a particular hospital. Belknap (1956) noted the alliance of the people we have called "Food and Shelter" with the custodial-oriented employees against the professional treatment personnel. There can occur what has been called the "edifice complex," an emphasis on buildings and equipment rather than the treatment of patients. For example, money may be "saved" and used to purchase new furniture. The wards "looked 100% better," something which is literally visible. Both adequate furniture and adequate professional staff are necessary in the treatment of psychiatric patients. It is a moot point which is more important when funds are limited.

Another matter which may be reflected by a high cost for food and shelter is the degree to which patients are employed to take a role in the hospital's maintenance and the degree to which they are taken care of within a traditional patient role. Mere number of hours or assignment to an activity will not reflect the degree that the work is meaningful and a preparation for extra-community adjustment. There can be elaborate assignments and programs to which patients do not come or in which they perform unnecessary activities. For future work, it seems reasonable to hypothesize that if meaningful participation is measured, it will be associated with reduced expenditure in the areas of food and shelter. However, if these activities are already overstaffed, the patient may model the idle employee.

## TREATMENT STAFF

The most interesting aspect of the findings dealing with treatment staff is the differential reflection in measures of effectiveness of the activities in which various professions engage. One of the most important findings of the present work is that the major impact of increased treatment staffing is reflected in the long hospitalization rather than the early release measure of effectiveness. This is paralleled by the finding in Table 16 that the greatest percentage difference in early FSR between favored ("good") and unfavored ("bad") hospitals was with the group with the poorest prognosis, the patients over 46 who had never married. With both measures of effectiveness, the greatest return is with the least "hopeful" cases. These data are not consistent with the current practice of the most intensive treatment being devoted to the newly admitted patient. These data also are at variance with the Joint Commission on Mental Illness and Health who distinguish between small, intensive treatment centers for patients with acute psychiatric illness and good prospect for improvement and the care of chronic psychiatric patients in existing State hospitals with more than 1000 beds (Joint Commission on Mental Illness and Health, 1961, pp. 266–8).

> We believe, however, that the final cost of treatment for the chronic patients would remain substantially below that of caring for the acutely ill patients who require intensive psychiatric treatment. Combined chronic disease hospitals could be operated at a great saving in professional personnel, particularly in skilled psychiatrists, psychologists and social workers of advanced degree and training who can more effectively work in intensive treatment centers (Joint Commission on Mental Illness and Health, 1961, p. 270).

Parallel to the finding that small size is associated with high percentage of early release while high staffing is associated with a low percentage of patients with long hospitalization, are the findings dealing with specific professional staff elements. The decision to discharge is a crucial aspect of rapid release. In this regard, the professional group most favorably associated with a high early release are the physicians who have administrative responsibility for releasing patients. It is interesting that a high percentage of the treatment staff devoted to PMR workers is negatively associated with a high percentage of early release. Contrasting physicians and PMR workers, we may hypothesize that the focus of the latter is on comfort and adjustment *within* the hospital while the former is the amelioration of symptomatic behavior and hence, for newly admitted patients, discharge. The professional group with the greatest impact on long hospitalization are social workers. This group, particularly through the home care program which is in their jurisdiction, paves the way for placement outside the hospital. In terms of special programs, it is interesting that the psychiatric residency and psychology trainee programs are significantly associated with a low percentage of patients with long hospitalization. Trainees are oriented towards treatment, professional goals, and in their student roles, frequently spend a greater amount of time with the professional literature and patients than do staff members who have supervisory and administrative duties.

Contrasting the professional groups and programs whose association with effectiveness seems to be favorable from those with random or negative favorability, we may return to our earlier formulation of minimal therapeutic requirements: there should be (a) maximum contact with patients by (b) people oriented towards returning them to the community. What is done for patients is quite directly reflected in the measures of effectiveness. Perhaps one of the most important findings of this work was this very specificity reflected, for example, in the significant correlation between the family care program and a lower percentage of patients with long hospitalization, and the random correlation between the family care program and early release. The difference between these correlations is all the more important when it is remembered that early release and long hospitalization are significantly correlated with each other.

## APPLICATIONS PER SIZE

The major points to be made about this variable may be found in the discussion of funding and displacement in the previous chapter. The more applications received for each bed, the higher was the early release rate and the lower was the percentage of patients with long hospitalization. Such a pressure of new patients provides a force towards discharge.

## SUMMARY

In this chapter the results were discussed in terms of the hospital milieu described in the previous chapter. Two generalizations seem plausible: other things being equal, people will engage in the activities that are most likely to lead to reinforcement, and these behaviors will be reflected, with surprising specificity, in differential measures of effectiveness.

## CHAPTER 11

# *Suggestions for Improvement*

WE HAVE discussed the behavior of both patients and employees as a function of the role enactments reinforced in the hospital situation. While the picture we have drawn may seem pessimistic, it is a picture of the strength of environmental influences, or, in the words of Arlidge quoted in the overview of this book, the degree to which "unpromising materials . . . may be drilled into order and guided by rule." If we can change the environment, hopefully we will be able to change the results we obtain. This chapter is devoted to ideas that may increase the effectiveness of psychiatric hospitals at little if any additional expense. The first section of this chapter will review suggestions drawn from Victor Thompson's *Modern Organization* (1963). This will be done in order to emphasize that Veterans Administration hospitals are *not* unique, but share problems common to most large contemporary organizations.

## THOMPSON'S SUGGESTIONS

To quote Thompson (1963, p. 195):

> In the first place, it might be wise to give most persons in supervisory positions some specific instrumental functions in addition to the exercise of authority, such as the factory foreman and the college-department chairman have. Not only would this practice keep the supervisor so busy that he would be forced to forego close supervision; but it would keep him also in touch with the technical realities and interdependencies of the organization.

At this point, Thompson remarks in a footnote that others have made similar suggestions such as increasing the number of supervisees in order to keep the supervisor busier and to reduce the supervisory salary bill.

Applying this suggestion to the psychiatric hospital, we can see that it increases the personnel who interact with patients as well as the supervisor's information about the treatment situation. In addition, a limited amount of staff time is available. This time may be used in staff–patient contact or staff–staff contact. It is not a question of whether one procedure is "good" and the other "bad," but how much of each will be of most benefit to patients. By placing the supervisor in the work situation part of the time, his opportunity to talk with employees is likely to be reduced to the point where it will be used for task-oriented purposes. Another way of stating this is that this suggestion is a remedy for the effect known as Parkinson's (first) law: that work expands so as to fill the time available for its completion. The supervisor who has time available will fill it by supervising his employees, an activity which keeps him busy and them away from patients.

To continue (Thompson, 1963, p. 195): "Secondly, a beginning might be made in the redefinition of 'success' if organizations were to establish two equal salary scales, one for specialists and one for the hierarchy." Thompson notes (1963, p. 196) that "Such a dual salary schedule would occasionally result in a situation (demolishing to status!) where the superior earns less than the subordinate." I personally would go further and suggest, as has Etzioni (1959, p. 67) ". . . in professional organizations staff and line concepts, to the degree that they can be applied at all, have to be reversed. The major (line) goal activity is carried out by experts." Much of an administrator's work can be done (and frequently is) by an intelligent secretary. Such a change in the reward system would have a salubrious effect in emphasizing more productive values and reducing extraneous political maneuvers. It would also do much to solve the paradox which was described by Belknap (1956, p. 68):

> A characteristic of this total system is that the levels with the most authority, training, and prestige are the farthest removed from the patient population in the hospital in terms of daily individual contact, and administrative work is the most heavily concentrated on those positions in the system which also carry the greatest medical and psychiatric responsibility for treating the patient.

A third point made by Thompson (1963, p. 196) is that "Wherever machine technology allows, the microdivision of labor should be ended. No longer should we throw a large part of the man away." When ancillary professions, secretaries, etc., are placed in supervisory hierarchies outside the province of the people who have responsibility for their work there is an unnecessary centralization which adds needless supervision by people unfamiliar with the work situation and deprives the person who assigns the work of effective control. Another aspect of the point raised by Thompson is that nurses, social workers, or psychologists, as well as psychiatrists, might be given prime responsibility for specific patients. This is suggested because interpersonal skills, particularly interviewing, are the common property of many professions. Next, responsibility and personal investment in their own cases (i.e. "*my* patient" rather than "a patient on Ward Eight–C") may lead to the personal involvement so severely lacking in bureaucratic settings. Schein (1965, p. 32) discusses this concept as an example of "job enlargement" in contrast to "job simplification." Henry (1957, p. 85) notes that, "The splitting of the task into several parts, each assigned to a different department, creates social distance between the executor of the task and the *directive force*, and between the executor of the task and the *task object*." Henry describes the use of "simple undifferentiated subordination" in which nearly complete responsibility for the patient is given the "counselor" and she is granted an enormous amount of autonomy and authority.

At present, there are many people who can veto therapeutic plans and who must be endlessly consulted within a bureaucratic system. If there should be anything that is grade enhancing, it should be responsibility in meeting the ostensible goals of the institution. The psychiatrist in charge of a ward should become a "functional foreman." If monetary considerations or the infrequent use of a speciality prevail, then there might be several functional foremen, ward psychiatrists, for whom the person works on special projects, patients. Thompson (1963, p. 104) discusses this matter and notes that this concept has never gained favor with management because it strikes at the very heart of the monocratic nature of the institution of hierarchy.

A fourth suggestion by Thompson (1963, pp. 196–7) is that:

> Specialist interdependencies created by acts of authority rather than by advance of specialization should be abolished. [Thompson remarks in a footnote that he refers to delegations resulting from power plays, from managerial esthetic needs for uniformity, etc.] Necessary interdependencies can themselves be hard to tolerate, but unnecessary ones are intolerable. In this connection it should be remembered that specialty depends upon an existing body of technique or knowledge which the individual masters by training and practice. If such a body of knowledge or technique does not exist, naming someone a specialist in such technique or knowledge does not make him one. True specialties cannot be created by acts of authority, but only by practice. . . . We are saying, in effect, that there should be decentralization wherever centralization cannot be shown to be necessary.

We have touched on this point in a number of ways. If the burden of proof passes to the hierarchy, and if pseudo-jargons and pseudo-statuses are placed under constant intelligent scrutiny, appreciable gains may be made in the organizational and professional climate of the hospital.

## SUGGESTIONS SPECIFIC TO THE PRESENT STUDY

In this section we will follow the general outline of the topics discussed in the previous three chapters.

### *The basis of funding*

In Chapter 9 it was pointed out that the use of the measure of average daily patient load emphasized in the very basis of funding a custodial rather than treatment goal. Alternatives to the use of average daily patient load are measures of turnover, size of the general population served, or, given the stability of turnover measures from year to year, improvement over previous reports of percentages of patients with long hospitalization. The same pressures which currently exist to maintain the proper level of patients *in* the hospital (as reflected in our quotation from Kennard, 1957) might be reversed and used to achieve the goal of discharge.

### *The need and availability of measures*

A general goal at the instrumental level is adequacy; Etzioni (1964, pp. 30–31) suggests "that organizations seek a *satisfying* solution rather than an optimum one. This means that search behavior will be stopped once a pattern is found which is considered 'reasonably good,' 'acceptable.' "

The problem becomes "what is reasonably good?" "what is acceptable?" This question indicates two important generalizations. First, there must be clarity of purpose at the very highest administrative levels as to what should be achieved. Second, there must be public, quantitative, reliable measures of the degree to which this goal has been attained. One of the accomplishments of the present work is the validation of routinely collected data (see the second preliminary study reported in Chapter 5). The method is developed, the material obtainable, and the additional expense of implementation negligible. What is required is an administrative decision to reinforce, with attention, prestige, and additional funds, progress along these lines. The material cited from Francis and Stone (1956) and Blau (1963) indicates how statistical records may be one mechanism for control.

### *Size*

Small size has a direct effect on patient treatment. Some of the favorable aspects of a small organization can be obtained if *functional* parts of the organization, wards and groups of wards, are decentralized into what is called the unit system (see Brill *et al.*, 1963, and Pepper, 1963, for descriptive details). A first benefit is that ideally the patient has the same staff during any one admission and during consecutive admissions. This permits a body of knowledge to develop, on the part of *both* staff and patients, which does not need to be started anew repeatedly. Such information and personal relationships are among the most crucial aspects of psychiatric treatment: they include confidence and ability to communicate on the part of patients, and knowledge of past history and indications of improvement on the part of the treatment staff. There is a decrease of time spent in reading and creating records.

A second advantage of the unit system lies in the decreased opportunity for the treatment staff to avoid responsibility by passing on its failures to "back wards" or "Siberias." While units may be large enough to permit some grading of wards such that psychological progress may be reinforced by literal "movement," the physician cannot forget his failures because they remain with him. The psychiatrist must deal with the patient who most requires his ministrations rather than sending him to a ward which is less well staffed. If confidence in success and expectation of improvement are important, it is difficult to think of anything less therapeutic than the validation of hopelessness caused by transfer to a chronic ward.

It is probable that heterogeneity of patient population is valuable. For the more severely maladjusted patient heterogeneity provides models with whom he can identify and whose behavior he can imitate. Fellow patients whose condition is less severe may provide clear examples of the behavior which will be reinforced by the staff. There is an assumption in this idea that the more severely disordered patients will model patients whose condition is less severe: it is presumed that adjustive behavior will be rewarded by the ward personnel. If the most withdrawn or delusional patient receives the most attention and tender loving care, we would expect that heterogeneity of patients would not be therapeutically beneficial. We shall return to this in our suggestions for nursing assistants. Cameron (1963) talked of homogeneity as follows: "If you want to help avoid dependent and regressed behavior, don't put patients liable to this type of behavior in a ward full of other dependent or regressed patients."

Finally, it should be noted that a unit system provides the benefits of smaller organizations in the work dealing with treatment while maintaining the advantages of large size for repetitive, impersonal, support functions such as the preparation of meals, payroll, and the like.

### *Applications per size*

The number of new applications received per unit size (bed) was favorably associated with both the early release and long hospitalization measures. Applications provide a pressure from outside the hospital for the discharge of patients. In a related manner, the number of patients beyond the level established as the hospital's average daily patient load provides a pressure for discharge. It may therefore be suggested that the hospital's average daily patient load be reduced by the organization's central office. In part, this is a step toward smaller size, but mainly it is a suggestion aimed at increasing the proportion of new applicants per bed and thus increasing pressure to free beds through rapid release and movement of long-term patients. Where the number of new applicants falls below a certain minimum (I would tentatively propose 75% of the ADPL per year), the ADPL should be cut.

This suggestion may seem inhumane. I think, however, that it is more in keeping with the purposes of society to seek for alternatives to hospitalization rather than to increase the number of hospital beds (Moore *et al.*, 1962). In line with this is the comment made by

Frank (1961, pp. 6–7) that social attitudes play such a big role in the definition of mental illness that people may be taught to consider normal reactions to stress as signs of mental illness: "The greater the number of treatment facilities and the more widely they are known, the larger the number of persons seeking their help. Psychotherapy is the only form of treatment which, at least to some extent, appears to create the illness it treats." Once a bed is available, there is a pressure to fill it. This circumstance is not unique to either the VA or the psychiatric professions, but may be a general aspect of normative organizations (Sills, 1961).

In keeping with funding for the purposes of society, the hospital might well be given additional staff in proportion to the number of applicants *not* admitted but for whom alternatives to hospitalization were found. In this manner an extra-hospital community orientation and an increasingly strong outpatient treatment service might be developed.

### *Allocation of funds within the hospital*

A major finding was that as the total *per diem* increased, the expense of all areas of hospital activity increased. The data for expenditures within the organization are routinely collected and reported. A single person with a desk calculator and piece of graph paper, if he were in a position to pursue specific expenditures and question excuses, could be of great benefit to the VA. As long as funds are limited, money spent on food and shelter means money not spent for treatment personnel. While food and shelter must be adequate, it is right, proper, and necessary to ask why one hospital spent $3.07 per patient per day while another spent $5.62 on the same services. Was the provision of food and shelter at the first hospital inadequate or is it possible that tighter administrative control could have increased the number of employees involved in the treatment of patients?

We have noted how Registrar services are ones which support the treatment aims of the hospital while the work done by Personnel deals with organizational functions. A first suggestion is that the emphasis in the allocation of funds be for services which facilitate and conserve the work of treatment personnel. A second suggestion harkens back to a definition of what behavior should be reinforced:

we noted in Chapter 9 that a bureaucrat's salary increased if he increased the number of employees he supervised. The purpose of the organization is not the supervision of employees. It is the accomplishment of a task. It would therefore seem to be more reasonable to increase the salary of workers in the area of general administration on the basis of decreasing the number of people required to provide a given service. This might be done in terms of a decreased number of office employees per patient, a decrease in employees over previous years, a decrease in time between initiation and completion of an action, or an increased number of *necessary* actions completed per employee. The word "necessary" has been underlined because if care is not taken, a situation similar to the example from Russia with which we concluded the ninth chapter is likely to occur: unnecessary actions which can be counted will accumulate. Whatever method is used, the goal should be the reinforcement of competence.

### *Treatment personnel*

The effectiveness of the treatment staff might be improved in much the same way as a monkey pounding on a typewriter can be helped to duplicate the works of Shakespeare. That is, we can increase the hours the monkey types (i.e. reinforce time with patients and decrease administrative ventures), or increase the number of monkeys engaged in typing (i.e. increase treatment staff through increased or more selective expenditures). However, even as with the monkeys, someone would be required to separate the poetry from the meaningless letters. While there is some value to "more of the same," the addition of something new seems called for.

A first suggestion in this area is that there be an increased interest and staffing of the chronic wards. This suggestion stems directly from the highly significant correlation between high treatment staff per patient and a low percentage of patients with long hospitalization. Continuing with our data, there should be increased emphasis and support of special programs such as family care placement which focus directly on the movement of long-term patients to the extra-hospital community.

A second suggestion deals with the area of nursing care. The concept of job enlargement applies to nurses and nursing assistants as much as it does to psychologists and social workers. Nursing assistants should be encouraged, trained, and rewarded for interacting with patients in a manner helpful to the achievement of the goal of returning patients to the community. While emphasis on a medical model does much to mitigate inhumane treatment, it is debatable whether considering the patient as sick and the object of uncritical benevolence is the best therapeutic course. On the one hand, the aide may have difficulty in understanding these concepts, and on the other, he may run into both technical and administrative difficulties if he applies them. Rather, nursing assistants should be taught to use reinforcers available to them contingent upon the patient emitting more adaptive behaviors. This concept parallels our remarks about the organization: a first step is a decision as to the overt, reliably identified behaviors that should be increased or used to replace undesirable or maladaptive behaviors. The next step is the identification of a reinforcing stimulus, a change in the environment which is meaningful to the person as defined by his altering his behavior to increase or decrease its presence. Finally, throughout this procedure, there is measurement to indicate the amount of progress. Failure is soon manifest in such a situation and indicates the need to alter the focal behaviors, the reinforcing stimulus, or the schedule of reinforcement. In such a procedure, as with organizational changes relevant to employees, care must be taken that the behavior wanted is the one reinforced. This topic is fully discussed and many case illustrations presented in Ullmann and Krasner (1965). The major issue at this point is that the nursing assistant be given explicit guidance in the positive things he can do. It is not sufficient either to tell him what patients should not do or to give him general psychodynamic principles. This is as unfair as it is to tell a patient to "get better" without delineating what "getting better" involves or making his changed behavior worthwhile.

We have mentioned the lack of power the functional leader (usually a psychiatrist) had within the bureaucratic system. Our earlier suggestions following Thompson (1963) imply an increase in the psychiatrist's authority to assign work, evaluate its performance, and if necessary, impose sanctions. Beyond the change involved in the current administrative lines by this suggestion, there is a very sensitive professional argument. Many of the most intelligent, active, and admirable staff and resident psychiatrists enter private practice, so that the psychiatrists who persevere and adjust to the institutional setting are not always ideal supervisors. I think, however, the crucial point lies in the selection of people who choose to remain in the system and adjust to it. After office expenses and taxes, the advantage in take home pay for a private psychiatrist is not so great that many outstanding men would not prefer the security, regular hours, companionship and professional rewards of hospital work.

Stone (1958, p. 496) summarizes a key issue when he writes: "Prestige for the professional becomes much the same as profit for the businessman." We have noted that professional prestige was undermined by a bureaucratic model, and it is therefore proposed that professional prestige and power be increased. In terms of role relations among professional people, the work of Zander, Cohen, and Stotland (1957) offers a number of valuable insights. The data for the Zander *et al.* study were obtained by means of individual interviews with 156 psychiatrists, 165 clinical psychologists, and 159 psychiatric social workers. A repeated finding was that the more powerful a psychiatrist perceived himself to be, the greater was his willingness to decrease his own power and to increase that of other professional groups. People seek contact with those who will facilitate their work and avoid those who hinder it; people who perceive their authority as secure are more liable to delegate responsibility than those whose security is threatened or non-existent. Zander *et al.* (1957, pp. 142–52) outline the inter-role strategies of superiors and subordinates. The cycle at present is vicious; by giving psychiatrists and other treatment personnel a clear objective, responsibility and prestige, it may become benign.

## THE HOSPITAL ADMINISTRATOR AS LOCUS OF CHANGE

The hospital director stands between the policy makers of the organization and the treatment employees. He may draw strength from both directions or he may draw fire from both. While the broad changes of policy and funding must be on a system-wide basis, there is much that the chief administrative officer at the hospital can do.

The director must be a diagnostician of the specific difficulties and opportunities in the hospital. He can allocate funds to specific services so that there is an emphasis on the purposes of the organization.

He can provide a personal example in a manner which the organization's central office cannot. He is, in Katz and Lazarsfeld's (1955) words, the "opinion leader." As such, his actions make manifest the concepts embodied in directives.

As has been pointed out previously in this book and by Argyris (1957) and McGregor (1960), employees learn to do what the organization expects of them. We have refined this in Chapter 9 to the formulation that employees' behavior reflects the behaviors for which they are reinforced. A good illustration of this in an industrial setting may be found in Gouldner's *Patterns of Industrial Bureaucracy* (1954) in which the new manager's assigned task leads him to perform in a manner different from his predecessor. In the area of psychiatric hospitals, Stotland and Kobler (1965) present a clear picture of the need for goals and the influence of the hospital director. Stotland and Kobler's work is all the more germane because the Director's employers, the Board, were not themselves clear as to the goals of the institution. Different Directors were interested in different goals with unfortunate results.

Much of the director's work occurs in small group meetings. Given a clear objective, the director must diagnose the behavior of group members. In this regard, it is well worth noting that activity, task ability, and likability tend to be randomly correlated with each other (Bales, 1958). The director may do well to identify each of these behaviors in the service chiefs with whom he meets and selectively reinforce (through attention, praise, and enactment) those behaviors he deems most useful in the attainment of his objectives. A second matter is that contrary to much of the literature, both popular and quasi-professional, there is no single most useful pattern of leadership. The situation and problem determine what interpersonal pattern will be most useful. Fiedler (1965), from a study of 53 sets of groups involving a total of over 800 separate groups, found that managing, controlling, directive leaders perform most effectively under either very favorable or very unfavorable situations. Where the task is highly structured permissive attitudes may obscure and delay necessary action. Where there is an extremely ambiguous situation, a directive chairman may be the most effective: once a reasonable decision has been made, it can be acted upon and such activity is likely to be more useful than continued inactivity. Permissive, accepting leaders would seem to be most effective when either they are personally disliked and therefore must be diplomatic or the task is an unstructured, creative one in which the cooperation of group members is needed. The hospital director should be able to identify the situations and shift his behavior according to the types of problems he encounters.

The hospital director is as much a therapist creating environments to alter behavior as is a therapist working with patients on the psychiatric ward. It is up to the director to make full use of the range of environmental resources at his command. Change in the hospital situation is most likely to occur through leadership from the top of the hierarchy down rather than from lower echelons up because, "Persons in a dependent position are by definition less able to initiate such action and to create an accepting climate for change" (Zander *et al.*, 1957, p. 153). Even more than the behavior therapist, however, the hospital director must be prepared to withstand counter-manipulation by the people whose behavior he wishes to alter. He must be prepared to deny reinforcement and extinguish activities that have previously been rewarded. Standing between the organization's policy makers and the hospital employees, the director has a difficult, thankless task, but if he does not carry it out, it is unlikely that anyone else will be able to.

## SUMMARY

This chapter presented suggestions for increasing the effectiveness of large, public psychiatric hospitals. The suggestions involved changes in supervisory activity, enlargement of the jobs of treatment employees, changes in the basis of funding to emphasize treatment rather than custodial objectives, the use of the unit system, reduction of hospital size to increase pressures for discharge, measurement and follow-up of the distribution of funds, promotion based on efficiency rather than number of employees supervised, staffing and special programs related to areas where they will have maximum impact, a focus particularly by aides on overt behaviors necessary for extra-community adjustment, and increased power and prestige for functional supervisors such as psychiatrists. Finally, the difficult but very crucial role played by the hospital director was discussed. While increased funds would be beneficial, these suggestions have avoided a concept of "more of the same" and endeavored to describe a more effective use of already available resources.

## CHAPTER 12

# *Summary*

THIS work started with the concept of an organization as a group of people with a common purpose. This purpose justifies the organization's existence and it is through the measurement of its attainment that the organization must be evaluated. We argued that the purpose of the psychiatric hospital is the return of patients to the community. The interpersonal difficulties of psychiatric patients were formulated in a sociopsychological model in order to designate the activities to be fostered in the hospital.

People are hospitalized when their behavior imposes inconvenience, embarrassment or suffering upon themselves or others. Social behavior rather than disease is the focus of psychiatric treatment and (Jackson, 1964, p. 45), "although the diagnostic categories employed may be psychiatric, the symptoms from which illness is inferred relate to social behavior." While other criteria were discussed, the purpose selected to evaluate hospitals was the return of patients to the community. Operationally, the measures of hospital effectiveness became (a) the percentage of newly admitted schizophrenics who returned to the community for at least 90 days within 274 calendar days after admission, and (b) the percentage of patients remaining in the hospital two or more years.

The problem then was to delineate the variables which would (a) increase early release and (b) decrease long hospitalization. From the course taken by the system of hospitals studied, from a review of the trends in psychiatric hospitals during the last 150 years, from the opinion of experts in the field, and from a review of literature in sociology and industrial psychology, two broad hypotheses were derived: small size and high staffing would be favorably associated with the effectiveness of psychiatric hospitals.

The major empirical results of the present work were the development and validation of measures of effectiveness and the delineation of the correlation between these criteria and various hospital characteristics. It was found that small size and high staffing were indeed favorably associated with effectiveness. Of greater importance, however, was that the data permitted a refinement of these statements into more explicit relationships. Chapter 8 provides a summary of the most striking relationships obtained and will not be repeated here. These results might be summarized by noting that for 30 hospitals a multiple correlation of .61 was derived for percentage of early release and a multiple correlation of .85 was derived for percentage of patients with long hospitalization. Two general findings deserve particular mention. The first was the specificity of relationships between certain hospital characteristics and the criteria of effectiveness. The second was the finding, somewhat at variance with the report of the Joint Commission on Mental Illness and Health (1961), that perhaps the greatest pay-off for small size and high staffing was with patients with the poorest prognosis.

In discussing the results, the hospital employee's day-to-day situation and accommodations were described. On a general level, it was proposed that a bureaucratic model is an inappropriate one for psychiatric hospitals. At a more specific level, it was argued that just as the behavior of psychiatric patients is a function of the actions reinforced within the social environment, so the employee's behavior is the reasonable outcome of the behavior reinforced within the environment to which he adjusts. The behavior of both patients and employees may be described within the same framework and explained by the same principles. The behaviors emitted are the ones reinforced, and in terms of this, we indicated how the reinforcement systems of the hospitals studied fostered custodial care and displacement of goals.

On the basis of our theoretical orientation, results, descriptions, and discussions, we arrived at a number of suggestions. These suggestions were specific ways in which current resources could be more effectively used and did not rely on increased expenditures. Given some of the findings, such as the increase in all areas of expense when the basic allocation increased, it is even possible that selective funding and careful control may lead to improved treatment at decreased cost.

Throughout, we stressed that VA hospitals are not unique but share problems common to most large modern organizations. Just as patients and employees exemplify the same principles which link experience and later behavior, so the problems of these psychiatric hospitals may be reflected in the adjustments of other clients and employees such as students and teachers. We have stressed the need to decide on overt measures of the purpose of the organization, a delineation of behaviors likely to lead to progress in achieving these purposes, and the reinforcement of such behaviors. In short, we presented (a) a functional analysis of behavior in the hospital situation for both patients and employees, and (b) data using psychological techniques for the study of individual differences among subjects, in this case 30 psychiatric hospitals.

Because psychiatric hospitals represent a major segment of clinical activity in terms of cost, number of patients, and involvement of professional staff, and because what happens within the hospital setting has definite ethical implications, the increased study and improvement of these institutions is imperative. In a broader sense, the psychiatric hospital is a small society unto itself and a valid laboratory for behavioral scientists concerned with bureaucratic organizations. The first aim of this work was applied in nature, as it should be with the human obligations involved. However, the treatment of hospitals as subjects and the utilization of the individual differences techniques and social learning theories developed by psychologists may be of value to political science, sociology, and anthropology beyond the purposes of a single governmental agency or a single problem area. Hopefully, this undertaking also has worthwhile implications for behavioral scientists as caretakers, citizens, and human beings struggling in the modern, organizational world.

# APPENDIX 1

## *Request for Information*

THIS study was made possible by the cooperation of the Veterans Administration Hospital Registrars, and very specifically, the good offices of Dr. H. Martin Engle, then Deputy Chief Medical Director of the Veterans Administration. The complete instructions for material from hospitals were transmitted in paragraph two of Department of Medicine and Surgery (DM&S) Circular 10–146 of August 7, 1961, which requested the submission of the following:

a. A list of all male patients admitted (including readmissions) to your hospital during fiscal years 1960 and 1961, i.e., between *July 1, 1959* and *June 30, 1961*. The list will be chronological and will include (1) the patient's name; (2) unit number; (3) date of admission; and (4) the admission diagnosis (item 33 of VA Form 10–2593). VA Form 7051, Data Sheet may be used for submitting this list in the original only.

b. A photocopy of both sides of the VA Form 10–2593, Record of Hospitalization, will be prepared for all male patients admitted during fiscal year 1960 (July 1, 1959 through June 30, 1960) for which the admission diagnosis was schizophrenic reaction of any type. (This includes photocopies of incomplete VA Forms 10–2593 on patients who were admitted in fiscal year 1960 and who remain on the hospital rolls.)

c. Prior to preparation of the photocopies all VA Forms 10–2593 will be checked to make sure that leaves of absence, trial visits and periods of elopement have been properly recorded. (This data will be recorded on the incomplete VA Forms 10–2593 submitted on patients who were admitted fiscal year 1960 and who remain on the hospital rolls.)

d. Photocopies of the two sides of each VA Form 10–2593 will be stapled together head to foot so that they will present the same appearance as the original document.

e. In those cases in which VA Form 10–2593 may not be available because a patient admitted in fiscal year 1960 was subsequently transferred, it is requested that a copy of the VA Form 10–2580 be submitted. The copy of the VA Form 10–2580 will contain the name of the hospital to which the patient was transferred.

APPENDIX 2

# *The VA Record of Hospitalization Form, SF 10–2593*

AS NOTED both in Appendix 1 and in the body of the text, the VA Record of Hospitalization form was a primary document in this study. At time of admission, completion of this form was started with such information as the veteran's name, identifying number at the hospital, his claim number, date of admission, permanent address, whom to notify in case of emergency, the relation to the veteran of this person, the veteran's date of birth, religion, marital status, occupation, branch of service, latest period of service, and admission diagnosis among other information useful either administratively or therapeutically. The first 35 items of the form were of this nature. Item 36A lists the *established clinical diagnoses* for which medical care was given. Item 36B asks for the designation of which one of the above (36A) diagnoses was primarily responsible for the major part of the patient's stay in the hospital. Item number 37 asks for other conditions, such as medical problems not treated or found only at autopsy. Items 38 and 39 deal respectively with operations performed at the hospital and special diagnostic and therapeutic procedures which might have been undertaken. Item 40 deals with compensation or pension status of the patient. Item number 41 deals with the disposition of the case, i.e. discharged, transferred, or died. Item number 42 is a place for the ward physician's signature and item 43 the date of disposition. Item number 44 was useful as a check as it asked for the number of inpatient days. Item 45 recapitulated briefly certain identifying information. Item 46 was of major importance in the present work since it gave a list of all leaves of absence (with or without permission) and trial visits. This material was entered by the specific dates of such leaves as well as the total days the patient was absent from the hospital. Item number 47 was a series of questions which comprised a medical certification of death. To summarize, the first 35 items yielded material by which to identify the patient, include him in the sample, and study the matter of sample correction. Items 36A and 36B were used in finding changes in diagnosis, and items 41, 44 and 46 in determining an early or late FSR.

## APPENDIX 3

# *Additional Material on Hospital Characteristics*

BECAUSE of the complexity of the material involved, to avoid further complication, presentation of data on the average, range, and stability over time was not included with the correlations dealing with differential staffing (Tables 10 *et seq.*). This Appendix may be considered a long footnote, or series of footnotes, presenting this material.

The range of *per diem* (money spent per patient per day) for *general administration*, was from $.94 to $1.83. The average amount spent on the area of general administration was $1.21. The product-moment correlation for the 30 hospitals between the expense per patient per day for general administration for fiscal years 1960 and 1961 was .97.

The range of *per diem* expense for the area of *non-nursing patient care* ranged for the 30 hospitals from $1.91 to $4.37. The average amount spent for non-nursing patient care per patient per day was $2.57. The correlation between the *per diem* expense for this area in fiscal year 1960 and fiscal year 1961 was .99.

The *per diem* expense for *nursing care* for the 30 hospitals ranged from $3.48 to $5.89. The average cost per patient per day for nursing care was $4.14. The correlation between expense in this area during fiscal year 1960 and fiscal year 1961 was .99.

The *per diem* expense for the area of *food and shelter* (Engineering, Dietetics, Housekeeping) ranged for the 30 hospitals from $3.07 to $5.62. The average cost per patient per day was $4.15. The correlation between successive years was .92.

It should be made explicit that the procedure was to compute the correlation between costs in successive years and after establishing the adequate stability of this characteristic, successive periods of time were averaged for each hospital. The figures used in correlations and reported in averages here therefore reflect averages of expenses during a two-year period.

No measure of stability over time was made for the next four measures since they were arrived at by simply dividing specific *per diem* expense by total *per diem* expense at each hospital. The *percentage* of total *per diem* for the area of general administration ranged from 8.8% to 12.0% with the average being 10.0%. The *percentage* of the total *per diem* spent on non-nursing patient care ranged from 17.4% to 25.3% with an average of 21.0%. The *percentage* of the total *per diem* spent on nursing care ranged from 30.3% to 39.7% with an average of 34.3%. The *percentage* of the total *per diem* spent for the area of food and shelter ranged from 29.3% to 39.8% with an average of 34.4%.

Across the 30 hospitals, the number of *physicians per 100 patients* ranged from .8 to 2.4 with an average of 1.44 per 100 patients. The correlation between physicians per 100 patients in fiscal years 1960 and 1961 was .89.

The number of *psychologists per 100 patients* ranged from .26 to 1.60 with an average of .63. The correlation between psychologists per 100 patients during fiscal year 1960 and fiscal year 1961 was .89.

The number of *social workers per 100 patients* ranged across the 30 hospitals from .22 to 1.96, with an average of .70. The correlation between social workers per 100 patients during fiscal year 1960 and fiscal year 1961 was .98.

The number of *physical medicine and rehabilitation workers* (PMR workers) *per 100 patients* ranged from 3.2 to 5.7 with an average of 4.12. The correlation between number of PMR workers per 100 patients during fiscal years 1960 and 1961 was .96.

The number of *nurses per 100 patients* ranged from 2.9 to 9.5, with an average of 5.44. The correlation between nurses per 100 patients during fiscal years 1960 and 1961 was .99.

The number of *nursing assistants per 100 patients* ranged from 21 to 35 with an average of 23.8. The correlation between number of nursing assistants per 100 patients during fiscal years 1960 and 1961 was .99.

As used in the present study, the number of treatment personnel per 100 patients was the sum, at each hospital, of the number of employees per 100 patients in each of the foregoing six categories (i.e., physicians, psychologists, social workers, PMR workers, nurses, and nursing assistants). The range of *treatment staff per 100 patients* across the 30 hospitals was from 30.2 to 54.2 with an average of 36.24. It is worth noting that the total number of employees per patient (FTE/ADPL) ranged from 59.4 to 114.5 per 100 patients with an average of 70.4 per 100 patients. In general, treatment personnel account for roughly half the hospital's employees.

No stability over time was computed for the next six characteristics since they simply involved dividing the number of personnel in each category by the total number of treatment personnel. This led to the percentage of treatment staff accounted for by each of the six types of employees. The *percentage* of the treatment staff composed of *physicians* ranged from 2.6% to 5.9% with an average of 3.97%. The *percentage* of the treatment staff composed of *psychologists* ranged from .7% to 3.1% with an average of 1.70%. The *percentage* of the treatment staff accounted for by *PMR workers* ranged from 9.0% to 15.0% with an average of 11.50%. The *percentage* of treatment staff accounted for by *nurses* ranged from 9.0% to 20.0% with an average of 14.87%. The *percentage* of treatment staff accounted for by *social workers* ranged from .7% to 3.1% with an average of 1.90%. The *percentage* of treatment staff accounted for by *nursing assistants* ranged from 60.0% to 73.0% with an average of 66.50%. While the purpose of this section is descriptive, this last figure, indicating that two-thirds of the treatment staff is composed of nursing assistants (aides, attendants) should be underlined. Further, members of this group of employees spend a far greater percentage of their duty time in direct patient contact than any other group of employees.

Ten of the hospitals had a *psychiatric residency* program during both years of the study; 14 of the hospitals had no such program in either year. The remaining six hospitals had a residency program one year, but not the next. A chi-square of 8.49, significant at the .01 level was obtained for presence or absence of the program in successive years and a score of one unit was assigned for each year such a program was in operation. The measure then became a residency program during zero, one or two years.

The number of *clinical psychology trainee* hours was obtained for the quarters ending in June 1959, 1960, and 1961, the beginning, middle, and end of the study period. These figures were divided by the size of the hospital (ADPL, average daily patient load) so that a measure of number of trainee hours per patient was obtained. From this, an estimate of trainee hours per patient per year was made across the 30 hospitals. The range was from .4 hours to 19.2 hours of psychology trainee time per patient per year, the average being 7.2. The correlations among number of trainee hours per patient for the three quarters ending in June which were used were as follows: between 1959 and 1960, .76; between 1959 and 1961, .75; between 1960 and 1961, .81. For purposes of the present work, the scores for the three quarters were averaged.

The amount of *research money* spent at each hospital during fiscal years 1960 and 1961 was divided by the number of patients. The correlation between the amount spent in these successive years was .79, the low correlation being due in major part to one hospital, already high in research funds, quadrupling its annual research budget. However, the 14 hospitals highest in research funds per patient and the 16 with the lowest amount of money spent on research did not change, so that a dichotomy could be made with no shifts from one year to the next (chi-square, one degree of freedom, of 22.75). Further, the highest amount spent at one of the 16 low research budget hospitals during the two years was $23. per patient, while the lowest amount spent at one of the 14 high research hospitals during the two years was $41. That is, the lowest "high" hospital spent 78% more than the highest "low" hospital. Across all hospitals, for the two year period, the range was from no expenditure (zero dollars per patient) to $289. per patient. To repeat, the score used was simply a dichotomous one, low or high.

The number of *family care placements* during the three calendar years, 1959, 1960, and 1961 were divided by the number of patients (size) of each hospital. The correlations among successive years for this measure of placements per patient were .95 between 1959 and 1960, .88 between 1959 and 1961, and .92 between 1960 and 1961. The placements per patient population during the three successive years were averaged to compose the score used in the present work. The range for this score was from .3 placements per thousand patients to 11.0 placements per thousand patients. The average hospital score was 2.42 placements per thousand patients per year.

The measure, *rural–urban* was simply a designation of the geographical area; it is worth keeping in mind when reading the material that a high numerical score is most rural (e.g. Fort Lyon, Colorado) and a low numerical score is most urban (e.g. VA hospitals in Pittsburgh and Los Angeles).

*New applications* are reported quarterly. The number of applicants at each hospital during the four quarters for fiscal years 1960 and 1961 were summed and divided by the patient population at each hospital. The correlation between figures for the two successive years was .98. The range for the 30 hospitals was from 25% to 209% with the number of applications received at the average hospital being 87.8% of the average daily patient load.

The range across 30 hospitals for *per diem* cost of *dietetics* was $1.68 to $2.43 with the average being $2.02. The correlation between *per diem* cost for dietetics in fiscal years 1960 and 1961 was .94.

The range of *per diem* cost for *engineering* was from $1.11 to $2.58 with the average being $1.72. The correlation between *per diem* cost in fiscal years 1960 and 1961 was .74.

The range of *per diem* cost for *housekeeping* was from $.19 to $.78 with the average being $.42. The correlation between *per diem* expenditure for housekeeping during fiscal years 1960 and 1961 was .96.

The *percentage* of the total *per diem* devoted to *dietetics* ranged from 13% to 21% with the average being 16.9%. The *percentage* of the total *per diem* devoted to *engineering* ranged from 11% to 19% with the average being 14.1%. The *percentage* of the total *per diem* devoted to *housekeeping* ranged from 1.6% to 5.4% with the average being 3.4%.

For the 30 hospitals, the range of *per diem* cost for the *office of the manager* ranged from $.040 to $.175 with an average of $.097. The correlation between *per diem* cost of the manager's office during fiscal years 1960 and 1961 was .91.

The *per diem* cost for *registrar's* services ranged from $.465 to $.840, the average being $.615. The correlation between cost of registrar during fiscal years 1960 and 1961 was .92.

The *per diem* cost for *fiscal* services ranged from $.120 to $.255 with an average of $.173. The correlation between *per diem* cost of fiscal service during fiscal years 1960 and 1961 was .96.

The *per diem* cost for the *personnel* office ranged from $.070 to $.180 with the average being $.106. The correlation between *per diem* cost of personnel during fiscal years 1960 and 1961 was .94.

The *per diem* cost for the *supply* office ranged from $.145 to $.305 with the average being $.210. The correlation between *per diem* expense for supply in fiscal year 1960 and fiscal year 1961 was .95.

The *percentage* of the total *per diem* devoted to the *office of the manager* ranged from .36% to 1.40% with the average being .79%. The *percentage* of the total *per diem* devoted to the *registrar's* office ranged from 4.4% to 6.2% with the average being 5.09%. The *percentage* of the total *per diem* devoted to the *fiscal* office ranged from 1.1% to 2.0% with the average being 1.43%. The *percentage* of the total *per diem* accounted for by the *personnel* office ranged from .66% to 1.07% with the average being .87%. The *percentage* of the total *per diem* accounted for by the *supply* office ranged from 1.3% to 2.4%, the average being 1.73%.

# *References*


ACTON SOCIETY TRUST (1953). *Size and morale: a preliminary study of attendance at work in large and small units.* London: AST.

ACTON SOCIETY TRUST (1957). *Size and morale: a further study of attendance at work in large and small units.* London: AST.

ALLPORT, F. (1933). *Institutional behavior.* Chapel Hill, N.C.: Univer. North Carolina Press.

AMERICAN PSYCHIATRIC ASSOCIATION (1952). *Diagnostic and statistical manual of mental disorders.* Washington, D.C.: Author.

ANDERSON, T. R., and WARKOV, S. (1961). Organizational size and functional complexity: a study of administration in hospitals. *Amer. Sociol. Rev.* **26,** 23–28.

ARGYRIS, C. (1956). *Diagnosing human relations in organizations.* New Haven, Conn.: Yale Univer. Labor and Management Center.

ARGYRIS, C. (1957). *Personality and organization.* New York: Harper.

ARLIDGE, J. T. (1859). *On the state of lunacy and the legal provision for the insane, with observations on the construction and organization of asylums.* London: John Churchill.

ATKINSON, R. L., and ROBINSON, N. M. (1961). Paired-associate learning by schizophrenic and normal subjects under conditions of personal and impersonal reward and punishment. *J. Abnorm. Soc. Psychol.* **62,** 322–6.

ATTHOWE, J. M., JR., and KRASNER, L. (1965). The systematic application of contingent reinforcement procedures (token economy) in a large social setting: a psychiatric ward. *Amer. Psychologist,* **20,** 591 (abstract).

AYLLON, T. (1963). Intensive treatment of psychotic behaviour by stimulus satiation and food reinforcement. *Behav. Res. Ther.* **1,** 53–61.

AYLLON, T., and AZRIN, N. H. (1965). The measurement and reinforcement of behavior of psychotics. *J. Exp. Anal. Behav.* **8,** 357–83.

AYLLON, T., and HAUGHTON, E. (1964). Modification of symptomatic verbal behaviour of mental patients. *Behav. Res. Ther.* **2,** 87–97.

AYLLON, T., and MICHAEL, J. (1959). The psychiatric nurse as a behavioral engineer. *J. Exp. Anal. Behav.* **2,** 323–34.

BABIGIAN, H. M., GARDNER, E. A., MILES, H. C., and ROMANO, J. (1965). Diagnostic consistency and change in a follow-up study of 1215 patients. *Amer. J. Psychiat.* **121,** 895–901.

BALINT, M. (1957). *The doctor, his patient, and the illness.* New York: International Univer. Press.

BALES, R. F. (1952). Some uniformities of behavior in small social systems. In G. SWANSON, T. NEWCOMB, and E. HARTLEY (Eds.) *Readings in social psychology.* New York: Holt, 146–59.

BALES, R. F. (1958). Task roles and social roles in problem-solving groups. In E. E. MACCOBY, T. M. NEWCOMB, and E. L. HARTLEY (Eds.) *Readings in social psychology* (3rd ed.). New York: Holt, Rinehart, Winston, 437–47.

BALES, R. F., and BORGATTA, E. F. (1955). Size of group as a factor in the interaction profile. In A. HARE, E. F. BORGATTA, and R. F. BALES (Eds.) *Small groups: studies in social interaction.* New York: Knopf, 396–413.

BANDURA, A. (1965). Behavioral modification through modeling procedures. In L. KRASNER and L. P. ULLMANN (Eds.) *Research in behavior modification.* New York: Holt, Rinehart, Winston, 310–40.

BARKER, R. G., and GUMP, P. V. (1964), in collaboration with BARKER, L. S., CAMPBELL, W. J., FRIESEN, W. V., HALL, E. R., LECOMPTE, W. F., and WILLEMS, E. P. *Big school, small school: high school size and student behavior.* Stanford, Calif.: Stanford Univer. Press.

BARR, A. (1958). Hospital size and staff sickness rates. *Brit. J. Prev. Soc. Med.* **12,** 156–8.

BARRABEE, P. S. (1951). A study of a mental hospital. Unpublished doctoral dissertation, Harvard Univer.

BARTON, R. (1959). *Institutional neurosis.* Bristol, England: Wright.

BASS, B. M., and NORTON, F. T. M. (1951). Group size and leaderless discussion. *J. Applied Psychol.* **35,** 397–400.

BAUMGARTEL, H., and SOBOL, R. (1959). Background and organizational factors in absenteeism. *Personnel Psychol.* **12,** 431–43.

BECK, A. T., WARD, C. H., MENDELSON, M., MOCK, J. E., and ERBAUGH, J. K. (1962). Reliability of psychiatric diagnoses: II. A study of consistency of clinical judgments and ratings. *Amer. J. Psychiat.* **119,** 351–7.

BECKER, H. S. (1963). *Outsiders.* New York: the Free Press of Glencoe.

BECKER, W. C. (1956). A genetic approach to the interpretation and evaluation of the process-reactive distinction in schizophrenia. *J. Abnorm. Soc. Psychol.* **53,** 229–36.

BELKNAP, I. (1956). *Human problems of a state mental hospital.* New York: McGraw-Hill, Blakiston Division.

BENDIX, R. (1956). *Work and authority in industry.* New York: Wiley.

BENNIS, W. G., BERKOWITZ, N., AFFINITO, M., and MALONE, M. (1958). Authority, power, and the ability to influence. *Hum. Relat.* **11,** 143–55.

BERNE, E. (1964). *Games people play.* New York: Grove Press (for the San Francisco Social Psychiatry Seminars).

BINDER, A. (1956). Schizophrenic intellectual impairment: uniform or differential? *J. Abnorm. Soc. Psychol.* **52,** 11–18.

BLAU, P. M. (1956). *Bureaucracy in modern society.* New York: Random House.

BLAU, P. M. (1963). *The dynamics of bureaucracy* (revised ed.). Chicago: Univer. of Chicago Press.

BLAU, P. M., and SCOTT, W. R. (1962). *Formal organizations.* San Francisco: Chandler.

BLOOM, S. W. (1963). *The doctor and his patient.* New York: Russell Sage Foundation.

BOCKOVEN, J. S. (1963). *Moral treatment in American psychiatry.* New York: Springer.

BRAYFIELD, A. H., and CROCKETT, W. H. (1955). Employee attitudes and employee performance. *Psychol. Bull.* **52,** 396–424.

BRIDGER, W. H. (1964). Contributions of conditioning principles to psychiatry. In *Pavlovian conditioning and American psychiatry* (GAP Symposium No. 9). New York: Group for the Advancement of Psychiatry, 181–98.

BRILL, H., FOLSOM, J., ST. PIERRE, R., and ZUBOWICZ, G. (1963). The unit system of operation. *Ment. Hosp.* **14,** 117–18.

BROMBERG, W. (1937). *The mind of man.* New York: Harper.

BROWN, G. W. (1960). Length of stay and schizophrenia: a review of statistical studies. *Acta Psychiat. Neurol. Scandinav.* **35,** 414–30.

Burling, T., Lentz, E. M., and Wilson, R. N. (1956). *The give and take in hospitals*. New York: Putnam.

Cameron, D. C. (1963). Patient-centered mental hospital administration. *The Unit Plan*. Conference transcript, Mental Health Association of Southeastern Pennsylvania (February 25, 1963). Published by Smith, Kline, & French.
Caplow, T. (1957). Organizational size. *Admin. Sci. Quart.* **1,** 484–505.
Castore, G. F. (1962). Number of verbal inter-relationships as a determinant of group size. *J. Abnorm. Soc. Psychol.* **64,** 456–8.
Caudill, W. (1956). Perspectives on administration in psychiatric hospitals. *Admin. Sci. Quart.* **1,** 155–70.
Caudill, W. (1958). *The psychiatric hospital as a small society*. Cambridge, Mass.: Harvard Univer. Press (Commonwealth Fund).
Clark, B. R. (1961). Organizational adaptation and precarious values. In A. Etzioni (Ed.) *Complex organizations*. New York: Holt, Rinehart, Winston, 159–67.
Cleland, S. (1955). *The influence of plant size on industrial relations*. Princeton, N.J.: Princeton Univer. Press.
Cohen, J. (1964). A rationale and method for psychiatric hospital assessment. In Symposium: An assessment of psychiatric hospital effectiveness. Amer. Psychol. Assoc. Convention, Los Angeles.
Cohen, J., and Struening, E. L. (1964). Opinions about mental health: hospital social atmosphere profiles and their relevance to effectiveness. *J. Consult. Psychol.* **28,** 291–8.
Cohen, R. A. (1957). Some relations between staff tensions and the psychotherapeutic process. In M. Greenblatt, D. J. Levinson, and R. H. Williams (Eds.) *The patient and the mental hospital*. Glencoe, Ill.: the Free Press, 301–8.
Coleman, J. C. (1956). *Abnormal psychology and modern life* (2nd ed.). Chicago: Scott, Foresman, & Co.
Cooley, C. H. (1909). *Social organization*. New York: Scribners.
Cooper, A. B., and Early, D. F. (1961). Evolution in the mental hospital: review of a hospital population. *Brit. Med. J.* June 3, 1600–3.
Cross, K. W., Harrington, J. A., and Mayer-Gross, W. (1957). A survey of chronic patients in a mental hospital. *J. Ment. Sci.* **103,** 146–71.
Cumming, E., and Cumming, J. (1956). The locus of power in a large mental hospital. *Psychiatry*, **19,** 361–9.
Cumming, J., and Cumming, E. (1957). Social equilibrium and social change in the large mental hospital. In M. Greenblatt, D. J. Levinson, and R. H. Williams (Eds.) *The patient and the mental hospital*. Glencoe, Ill.: the Free Press, 49–72.
Cumming, J., and Cumming, E. (1962). *Ego and milieu*. New York: Atherton Press.

Dain, N. (1964). *Concepts of insanity in the United States, 1789–1865*. New Brunswick, N.J.: Rutgers Univer. Press.
Dalton, M. (1959). *Men who manage*. New York: Wiley.
Davis, A. K. (1948). Bureaucratic patterns in the Navy Officer Corps. *Social Forces*, **27,** 143–53.
Davis, J. E. (1964). Empirical dimensions of psychiatric hospital organization. In Symposium: An assessment of psychiatric hospital effectiveness. Amer. Psychol. Assoc. Convention, Los Angeles.

DAVISON, G. C. (1965). The influence of systematic desensitization, relaxation, and graded exposure to imaginal aversive stimuli on the modification of phobic behavior. Unpublished doctoral dissertation, Stanford Univer., Stanford, Calif.

DAWE, H. C. (1934). The influence of size of kindergarten group upon performance. *Child Developm.* **5,** 295–303.

DEITER, J. B., HANFORD, D. B., HUMMEL, R. T., and LUBACH, J. E. (1964). A pilot hospital program applicable to treating major mental illness in community centers. Paper read at Western Psychol. Assoc. Convention, Portland, Ore.

DEUTSCH, A. (1946). *The mentally ill in America.* New York: Columbia Univer. Press.

DIMOCK, M. E. (1952). Bureaucracy self-examined. In R. K. MERTON, A. P. GRAY, B. HOCKEY, and H. C. SELVIN (Eds.) *Reader in bureaucracy.* Glencoe, Ill.: the Free Press, 397–406.

DUBIN, R. (1951). *Human relations in administration.* New York: Prentice-Hall.

DUNHAM, H. W., and WEINBERG, S. K. (1960). *The culture of the state mental hospital.* Detroit: Wayne State Univer. Press.

DURKHEIM, E. (1902). *De la division du travail social.* Paris: Felix Alcan.

ETZIONI, A. (1959). Authority structure and organizational effectiveness. *Admin. Sci. Quart.* **4,** 43–67.

ETZIONI, A. (1960a). Two approaches to organizational analysis: a critique and a suggestion. *Admin. Sci. Quart.* **5,** 257–78.

ETZIONI, A. (1960b). Interpersonal and structural factors in the study of mental hospitals. *Psychiatry,* **23,** 13–22.

ETZIONI, A. (Ed.) (1961). *Complex organizations.* New York: Holt, Rinehart, Winston.

ETZIONI, A. (1964). *Modern organizations.* Englewood Cliffs, N.J.: Prentice-Hall.

EXPERT COMMITTEE ON MENTAL HEALTH (1953). *Third Report.* Geneva: World Health Organization, Technical Reports, Series No. 73.

FARINA, A., GARMEZY, N., and BARRY, H., III. (1963). Relationship of marital status to incidence and prognosis of schizophrenia. *J. Abnorm. Soc. Psychol* **67,** 624–30.

FERSTER, C. B. (1958). Reinforcement and punishment in the control of human behavior by social agencies. *Psychiat. Res. Rep.* **10,** 101–18.

FERSTER, C. B. (1965). Classification of behavioral pathology. In L. KRASNER and L. P. ULLMANN (Eds.) *Research in behavior modification.* New York: Holt, Rinehart, Winston.

FIEDLER, F. E. (1965). The contingency model: a theory of leadership effectiveness. In H. PROSHANSKY and B. SEIDENBERG (Eds.) *Basic studies in social psychology.* New York: Holt, Rinehart, Winston, 538–51.

FRANCIS, R. G., and STONE, R. C. (1956). *Service and procedure in bureaucracy.* Minneapolis: Univer. Minnesota Press.

FRANK, J. D. (1961). *Persuasion and healing.* Baltimore: Johns Hopkins Press.

FREEMAN, H. (1958). The tranquilizing drugs. In L. BELLAK (Ed.) *Schizophrenia: a review of the syndrome.* New York: Logos Press, 473–500.

FREEMAN, H. E., and SIMMONS, O. G. (1961). Consensus and coalition in the release of mental patients. *Hum. Org.* **20,** 89–91.

FREEMAN, H. E., and SIMMONS, O. G. (1963). *The mental patient comes home*, New York: Wiley.
FREIDSON, E. (Ed.) (1963). *The hospital in modern society*. New York: the Free Press of Glencoe.
FREUDENBERG, R., and ROBERTSON, J. (1956). Symptoms in relation to psychiatric diagnosis and treatment. *Arch. Neurol. Psychiat.* **76,** 14–22.
FROMM, E. (1941). *Escape from freedom*. New York: Rinehart.
FROMM, E. (1947). *Man for himself*. New York: Rinehart.
FULLER, R. G. (1930). Expectation of hospital life and outcome for mental patients on first admission. *Psychiat. Quart.* **4,** 295–323.

GARDNER, B. B., and MOORE, D. G. (1952). *Human relations in industry*. Homewood, Ill.: R. D. Irwin.
GARRATT, F. N., LOWE, C. R., and MCKEOWN, T. (1958). Investigation of the medical and social needs of patients in mental hospitals. II. Type of accommodation and staff required. *Brit. J. Prev. Soc. Med.* **12,** 23–41.
GEORGOPOULOS, B. S., and MANN, F. C. (1962). *Community general hospital*. New York: Macmillan.
GINZBERG, E. (1949). *A pattern for hospital care*. New York: Columbia Univer. Press.
GIOVANNONI, J. M., and ULLMANN, L. P. (1961). Characteristics of family care homes. *Int. J. Soc. Psychiat.* **7,** 299–306.
GLASS, COL. (1957). In *Preventive and social psychiatry*. Washington, D.C.: U.S. Printing Office.
GOFFMAN, E. (1961). *Asylums*. Garden City, N.Y.: Doubleday Anchor Books.
GOLDSTEIN, A. (1962). *Therapist–patient expectancies in psychotherapy*. New York: Pergamon Press.
GOULDNER, A. W. (1952). Red tape as a social problem. In R. K. MERTON, A. P. GRAY, B. HOCKEY, and H. C. SELVIN (Eds.) *Reader in bureaucracy*. Glencoe, Ill.: the Free Press, 410–18.
GOULDNER, A. W. (1954). *Patterns of industrial bureaucracy*. Glencoe, Ill.: the Free Press.
GREENBLATT, M., YORK, R. H., and BROWN, E. L. (1955), in collaboration with HYDE, R. W. *From custodial to therapeutic patient care in mental hospitals*. New York: Russell Sage Foundation.
GUREL, L. (1964). Correlates of psychiatric hospital effectiveness. In Symposium: An assessment of psychiatric hospital effectiveness. Amer. Psychol. Assoc. Convention, Los Angeles.

HAMILTON, S. W. (1944). The history of American mental hospitals. In J. K. HALL (Ed.) *One hundred years of American psychiatry*. New York: Columbia Univer. Press, 73–166.
HARE, A. P. (1952). A study of interaction and consensus in different sized groups. *Amer. Sociol. Rev.* **17,** 261–7.
HARMS, E. (1957). Modern psychotherapy—150 years ago. *J. Ment. Sci.* **103,** 804–9.
HASTORF, A. H. (1965). The reinforcement of individual actions in a group situation. In L. KRASNER, and L. P. ULLMANN (Eds.) *Research in behavior modification*. New York: Holt, Rinehart, Winston, 271–84.
HAYES, K. J. (1962). Genes, drives, and intellect. *Psychol. Rep.* **10,** 299–342 (Monogr. Supp. 2-V10).

HEMPHILL, J. K. (1950). Relations between the size of the group and the behavior of "superior" leaders. *J. Soc. Psychol.* **32,** 11–22.

HENRY, J. (1954). The formal social structure of a psychiatric hospital. *Psychiatry,* **17,** 139–51.

HENRY, J. (1957). Types of institutional structure. In M. GREENBLATT, D. J. LEVINSON, and R. H. WILLIAMS, *The patient and the mental hospital.* Glencoe, Ill.: the Free Press, 73–90.

HENRY, J. (1964). Space and power in a psychiatric unit. In A. F. WESSEN (Ed.) *The psychiatric hospital as a social system.* Springfield, Ill.: Chas. C. Thomas, 20–34.

HESS, I., RIEDEL, D. C., and FITZPATRICK, T. B. (1961). *Probability sampling of hospitals and patients.* Ann Arbor: Univer. Michigan Press.

HEWITT, D., and PARFITT, J. (1953). A note on working morale and size of group. *Occupational Psychol.* **27,** 38–42.

HILGARD, E. R. (1956). *Theories of learning* (2nd ed.). New York: Appleton-Century-Crofts.

HOFFMAN, J. L. (1957). Problems of administration in a large mental hospital. In M. GREENBLATT, D. J. LEVINSON, and R. H. WILLIAMS (Eds.) *The patient and the mental hospital.* Glencoe, Ill.: the Free Press, 46–48.

HOLMES, D. J. (1964). *The adolescent in psychotherapy.* Boston: Little, Brown, & Co.

HONIGFELD, G. (1963). *The placebo effect: a review of non-specific factors in treatment.* Perry Point, Maryland: Central Neuropsychiatric Research Laboratory, Report No. 55.

HUNT, J. McV. (1961). *Intelligence and experience.* New York: Ronald Press.

HUNTER, R., and MACALPINE, I. (Eds.) (1963). *Three hundred years of psychiatry, 1535–1860.* London: Oxford Univer. Press.

HUTT, M. L., and GIBBY, R. G. (1957). *Patterns of abnormal behavior.* Boston: Allyn & Bacon.

HYDE, R. W., and WILLIAMS, R. H. (1957). What is therapy and who does it? In M. GREENBLATT, D. J. LEVINSON, and R. H. WILLIAMS (Eds.) *The patient and the mental hospital.* Glencoe, Ill.: the Free Press, 173–96.

INDIK, B. P. (1963). Some effects of organization size on member attitudes and behavior. *Hum. Relat.* **16,** 369–84.

INDIK, B. P. Organization size and member participation: some empirical tests of alternative explanations. *Hum. Relat.* (in press).

JACKSON, D. D. (Ed.) (1960). *The etiology of schizophrenia.* New York: Basic Books.

JACKSON, J. (1964). Toward the comparative study of mental hospitals: characteristics of the treatment environment. In A. F. WESSEN (Ed.) *The psychiatric hospital as a social system.* Springfield, Ill.: Chas. C. Thomas, 35–87.

JACO, E. G. (Ed.) (1958). *Patients, physicians, and illness.* Glencoe, Ill.: the Free Press.

JENKINS, R. L. (1961). A preliminary report on the Psychiatric Evaluation Project. *Coop. Stud. Psychiat. Res.* **6,** 361–6.

JENKINS, R. L., and GUREL, L. (1959). Predictive factors in early release. *Ment. Hosp.* **10** (Nov.), 11–14.

JOHNSON, R., and McNEAL, B. F. (1964). Combined MMPI and demographic data in predicting length of neuropsychiatric hospital stay. *J. Consult. Psychol.* **28,** 64–70.

JOINT COMMISSION ON MENTAL ILLNESS AND HEALTH (1961). *Action for mental health*. New York: Science Editions.

JONES, E. (1953). *The life and work of Sigmund Freud*. New York: Basic Books.

JONES, K. (1963). The role and function of the mental hospital. In H. FREEMAN and J. FARNDALE (Eds.) *Trends in the mental health services*. New York: Macmillan (a Pergamon Press Book), 60–71.

JONES, K., and SIDEBOTHAM, R. (1962). *Mental hospitals at work*. London: Routledge & Kegan Paul.

JONES, M. (1953). *The therapeutic community*. New York: Basic Books.

KAHNE, M. J. (1959). Bureaucratic structure and impersonal experience in mental hospitals. *Psychiatry*, **22,** 363–75.

KAMMAN, G. F., LUCERO, R. J., MEYER, B. T., and RECHTSCHAFFEN, A. (1954). Critical evaluation of a total push program for regressed schizophrenics in a state hospital. *Psychiat. Quart.* **28,** 650–67.

KATZ, E., and LAZARSFELD, P. F. (1955). *Personal influence*. Glencoe, Ill.: the Free Press.

KAUFMAN, L. N. (1964). The effects of interpersonal interaction on abstract thinking performance of schizophrenics. *Amer. Psychologist* **19,** 460 (abstract).

KELLEY, H. H., and THIBAUT, J. W. (1954). Experimental studies of group problem solving and process. In G. LINDZEY (Ed.) *Handbook of social psychology*. Cambridge, Mass.: Addison-Wesley, 735–85.

KELLY, E. L., and GOLDBERG, L. R. (1959). Correlates of later performance and specialization in psychology. *Psychol. Monogr.* **73,** No. 12 (whole No. 482).

KENDALL, P. L. (1963). The learning environment of hospitals. In E. FREIDSON (Ed.) *The hospital in modern society*. New York: the Free Press of Glencoe, 195–230.

KENNARD, E. A. (1957). Psychiatry, administrative psychiatry, administration: a study of a veterans hospital. In M. GREENBLATT, D. J. LEVINSON, and R. H. WILLIAMS (Eds.) *The patient and the mental hospital*. Glencoe, Ill.: the Free Press, 36–45.

KING, G. F., ARMITAGE, S. G., and TILTON, J. R. (1960). A therapeutic approach to schizophrenics of extreme pathology: an operant-interpersonal method. *J. Abnorm. Soc. Psychol.* **61,** 276–86.

KING, S. H. (1962). *Perceptions of illness and medical practice*. New York: Russell Sage Foundation.

KLUCKHOHN, C., and MURRAY, H. A. (Eds.) (1950). *Personality in nature, society, and culture*. New York: Knopf.

KRAEPELIN, E. (1962). *One hundred years of psychiatry*. (Translated by Wade Baskin.) New York: Citadel Press.

KRAMER, M., GOLDSTEIN, H., ISRAEL, R. H., and JOHNSON, N. A. (1955). *A historical study of the disposition of first admissions to a state mental hospital*. Public Health Monogr. No. 32, Washington: U.S. Govt. Printing Office.

KRASNER, L. (1958). Studies of the conditioning of verbal behavior. *Psychol. Bull.* **55,** 148–70.

KRASNER, L., and ULLMANN, L. P. (Eds.) (1965). *Research in behavior modification*. New York: Holt, Rinehart, Winston.

LAZARSFELD, P. F., and THIELENS, W., JR. (1958). *The academic mind*. Glencoe, Ill.: the Free Press.

LEAVITT, H. J. (1958). *Managerial psychology*. Chicago: Univer. of Chicago Press.

LEHRMAN, N. S. (1961). Do our hospitals help make acute schizophrenia chronic? *Dis. Nerv. Syst.* **22,** 489–93.

LEVINSON, D. J., and GALLAGHER, E. B. (1964). *Patienthood in the mental hospital.* Boston: Houghton Mifflin.

LEWIS, N. D. C. (1941). *A short history of psychiatric achievement.* New York: Norton.

LIEBERMAN, S. (1956). The effects of changes in roles on the attitudes of role occupants. *Hum. Relat.* **9,** 385–402.

LOEB, M. B. (1957). Role definition in the social world of a psychiatric hospital. In M. GREENBLATT, D. J. LEVINSON, and R. H. WILLIAMS (Eds.) *The patient and the mental hospital.* Glencoe, Ill.: the Free Press, 14–19.

MALZBERG, B. (1958). *Cohort studies of mental disease in New York State: 1943–1949.* New York: National Assoc. for Mental Health.

MARCH, J. G., and SIMON, H. A. (1958). *Organizations.* New York: Wiley.

MARRIOTT, R. (1949). Size of working group and output. *Occupational Psychol.* **23,** 47–57.

MCCARTHY, J. F. (1964). The differential effects of praise and censure upon the verbal responses of schizophrenics. *Amer. Psychologist,* **19,** 459 (abstract).

MCGAUGHRAN, L. S., and MORAN, L. J. (1956). "Conceptual level" vs. "conceptual area" analysis of object-sorting behavior of schizophrenic and non-psychiatric groups. *J. Abnorm. Soc. Psychol.* **52,** 43–50.

MCGREGOR, D. M. (1960). *The human side of enterprise.* New York: McGraw-Hill.

MCNEMAR, Q. (1962). *Psychological statistics* (3rd ed.). New York: Wiley.

MCREYNOLDS, P. (1960). Anxiety, perception, and schizophrenia. In D. D. JACKSON (Ed.) *The etiology of schizophrenia.* New York: Basic Books, 248–92.

MEICHENBAUM, D. H. (1965). The effects of social reinforcement on the level of abstraction in schizophrenics. Unpublished Masters Thesis, Univer. of Illinois.

MENNINGER, K. (1959). *A psychiatrist's world.* New York: Viking Press.

MENNINGER, K. (1964). Psychiatrists use dangerous words. *Saturday Evening Post,* **237** (No. 16, April 25), 12–14.

MERRIHUE, W. V., and KATZELL, R. A. (1955). ERI—yardstick of employee relations. *Harvard Bus. Rev.* **33** (6), 91–99.

MERTON, R. K. (1940). Bureaucratic structure and personality. *Social Forces,* **17,** 560–8.

MERTON, R. K., GRAY, A. P., HOCKEY, B., and SELVIN, H. C. (Eds.) (1952). *Reader in bureaucracy.* Glencoe, Ill.: the Free Press.

MERTON, R. K. (1957). *Social theory and social structure* (2nd ed.). Glencoe, Ill.: the Free Press.

METROPOLITAN COMMISSIONERS IN LUNACY (1844). *Report to the Lord Chancellor.* (Presented to both Houses of Parliament by command of Her Majesty.)

MILLER, G. A. (1957). Communication and information as limiting factors in group formation. In *Preventive and social psychiatry.* Washington, D.C.: U.S. Printing Office, 1–13.

MISHLER, E. G., and TROPP, A. (1956). Status and interaction in a psychiatric hospital. *Hum. Relat.* **9,** 187–205.

MISHLER, E. G., and WAXLER, N. E. (1963). Decision processes in psychiatric hospitalization: patients referred, accepted, and admitted to a psychiatric hospital. *Amer. Sociol. Rev.* **28,** 576–87.

MOORE, R. F., ALBERT, R. S., MANNING, M. J., and GLASSER, B. A. (1962). Explorations in alternatives to hospitalization. *Amer. J. Psychiat.* **119,** 560–9.

MOORE, W. E. (1951). *Industrial relations and the social order* (rev. ed.). New York: Macmillan.

MOORE, W. E. (1964). *The conduct of the corporation.* New York: Random House Vintage Books.

NORTON, A. (1961). Mental hospital ins and outs: a survey of patients admitted to a mental hospital in the past 30 years. *Brit. Med. J.* (2/25), 528–36.

ODEGARD, O. (1961). Pattern of discharge and readmission in psychiatric hospitals in Norway, 1926 to 1955. *Ment. Hyg.* **45,** 185–93.

ORNE, M. T. (1962). On the social psychology of the psychological experiment: with particular reference to demand characteristics and their implications. *Amer. Psychologist* **17,** 776–83.

ORNE, M. T., and SCHEIBE, K. E. (1964). The contribution of nondeprivation factors in the production of sensory deprivation effects: the psychology of the "panic button". *J. Abnorm. Soc. Psychol.* **68,** 3–12.

OZARIN, L. D. (1954). Moral treatment and the mental hospital. *Amer. J. Psychiat.* **111,** 371–8.

PAGE, C. H. (1946). Bureaucracy's other face. *Social Forces,* **25,** 88–94.

PARKINSON, C. N. (1957). *Parkinson's law.* Boston: Houghton Mifflin.

PARKINSON, C. N. (1960). *The law and the profits.* Boston: Houghton Mifflin.

PARKINSON, C. N. (1962). *In-laws and outlaws.* Boston: Houghton Mifflin.

PARSONS, T. (1951). *The social system.* Glencoe, Ill.: the Free Press.

PARSONS, T. (1957). The mental hospital as a type of organization. In M. GREENBLATT, D. J. LEVINSON, and R. H. WILLIAMS (Eds.) *The patient and the mental hospital.* Glencoe, Ill.: the Free Press, 108–29.

PASAMANICK, B., DINITZ, S., and LEFTON, M. (1959). Psychiatric orientation and its relation to diagnosis and treatment in a mental hospital. *Amer. J. Psychiat.* **116,** 127–32.

PAUL, G. L. (1964). Comparative psychotherapeutic effectiveness in the treatment of performance anxiety: stress condition results. Paper presented to Midwest. Psychol. Assoc.

PEPPER, M. P. (1963). Overview of practices. *The Unit Plan.* Conference transcript, Mental Health Assoc. of Southeastern Pennsylvania, February 25, 1963 (published by Smith, Kline, & French).

PERROW, C. (1965). Hospitals: technology, structure, and goals. In J. G. MARCH (Ed.) *Handbook of organizations.* Chicago: Rand McNally, 910–71.

PETERS, H. N., and JENKINS, R. L. (1954). Improvement of chronic schizophrenic patients with guided problem-solving, motivated by hunger. *Psychiat. Quart. Suppl.* **28,** 84–101.

PORTER, L. W., and LAWLER, E. E., III. (1956). Properties of organization structure in relation to job attitudes and job behavior. *Psychol. Bull.* **64,** 23–51.

POWELL, N. J. (1956). *Personnel administration in government.* Englewood-Cliffs, N.J.: Prentice-Hall.

PRESTHUS, R. (1962). *The organizational society.* New York: Knopf.

READER, G. E., and GOSS, M. E. W. (1959). Medical sociology with particular reference to the study of hospitals. *Transactions of the Fourth World Congress of Sociology*, Vol. 2, London: International Sociological Association, 139–52.

REES, T. P. (1957). Back to moral treatment and community care. *J. Ment. Sci.* **103,** 303–13.

REIMANIS, G. (1965a). Effects of a Veterans Administration Center closing announcement on member and patient behavior. *Newsletter Res. Psychol.* **7** (No. 4), 37–39.

REIMANIS, G. (1965b). Effects of future uncertainty on anomie. *Newsletter Res. Psychol.* **7** (No. 4), 39–40.

REVANS, R. W. (1957). Staff turnover—its causes and remedies. In *Hospital authorities and staff management.* London: Royal Institute of Public Administration, 34.

REVANS, R. W. (1958). Human relations, management, and size. In E. M. HUGH-JONES (Ed.) *Human relations and modern management.* Amsterdam, Netherlands: North Holland Publishing Co., 177–220.

RICKARD, H. C., DIGMAN, P. J., and HORNER, R. F. (1960). Verbal manipulation in a psychotherapeutic relationship. *J. Clin. Psychol.* **16,** 364–7.

RICKARD, H. C., and DINOFF, M. (1962). A follow-up note on "verbal manipulation in a psychotherapeutic relationship". *Psychol. Rep.* **11,** 506.

RIESMAN, D., GLAZER, N., and DENNEY, R. (1950). *The lonely crowd.* New Haven: Yale Univer. Press.

ROSENTHAL, R. (1963). On the social psychology of the psychological experiment: the experimenter's hypothesis as unintended determinant of experimental results. *Amer. Sci.* **51,** 268–82.

RUESCH, J. (1950). Social technique, social status, and social change in illness. In C. KLUCKHOHN and H. A. MURRAY (Eds.) *Personality in nature, society, and culture.* New York: Knopf, 117–30.

RUSHING, W. A. (1964). *The psychiatric professions.* Chapel Hill, N.C.: Univer. North Carolina Press.

SALZINGER, K., and PISONI, S. (1958). Reinforcement of affect responses of schizophrenics during the clinical interview. *J. Abnorm. Soc. Psychol.* **57,** 84–90.

SANDIFER, M. G., JR., PETTUS, C., and QUADE, D. (1964). A study of psychiatric diagnosis. *J. Nerv. Ment. Dis.* **139,** 350–6.

SCHACHTER, S., and SINGER, J. E. (1962). Cognitive, social, and physiological determinants of emotional state. *Psychol. Rev.* **69,** 379–99.

SCHEIN, E. H. (1965). *Organizational psychology.* Englewood Cliffs, N.J.: Prentice-Hall.

SCHEIN, E. H., with SCHNEIER, I., and BARKER, C. H. (1961). *Coercive persuasion.* New York: Norton.

SCHMIDT, H. O., and FONDA, C. P. (1956). The reliability of psychiatric diagnosis: a new look. *J. Abnorm. Soc. Psychol.* **52,** 262–7.

SCHWARTZ, M. (1957). What is a therapeutic milieu? In M. GREENBLATT, D. J. LEVINSON, and R. H. WILLIAMS (Eds.) *The patient and the mental hospital.* Glencoe, Ill.: the Free Press.

SCHWARTZ, M. S., and SCHWARTZ, C. G. (1964). *Social approaches to mental patient care.* New York: Columbia Univer. Press.

SCOTT, W. A. (1958). Research definitions of mental health and mental illness. *Psychol. Bull.* **55,** 29–45.

SEWALL, L., and BERGER, D. (1959). A medical audit plan for psychiatric hospitals. *Ment. Hosp.* **10,** 7–10.

SHAPIRO, A. K. (1960). A contribution to a history of the placebo effect. *Behav. Sci.* **5,** 109–35.

SHARP, W. R. (1952). Procedural vices: La Paperasserie. In R. K. MERTON, A. P. GRAY, B. HOCKEY, and H. C. SELVIN (Eds.) *Reader in bureaucracy.* Glencoe, Ill.: the Free Press, 407–10.

SIEGEL, S. (1956). *Nonparametric statistics for the behavioral sciences.* New York: McGraw-Hill.

SILLS, D. L. (1961). The succession of goals. In A. ETZIONI (Ed.) *Complex organizations.* New York: Holt, Rinehart, Winston, 146–59.

SIMMEL, G. (1902). The number of members as determining the sociological form of the group. *Amer. J. Sociol.* **8,** 1–196.

SIMON, H. A., SMITHBURG, D. W., and THOMPSON, V. A. (1959). *Public administration.* New York: Knopf.

SKINNER, B. F. (1953). *Science and human behavior.* New York: Macmillan.

SMITH, H. L. (1949). The sociological study of hospitals. Unpublished doctoral dissertation, Univer. of Chicago.

SMITH, H. L. (1955). Two lines of authority are one too many. *Modern Hosp.* **84** (No. 3, March), 59–64.

SOLOMON, D. N. (1957). Professional persons in bureaucratic organizations. In *Preventive and social psychiatry.* Washington, D.C.: U.S. Government Printing Office, 253–66.

SOLOMON, H. C. (1951). Treatment of the psychoses. *Psychiat. Quart.* **25,** 1–19.

SOMMER, R., and OSMOND, H. (1961). Symptoms of institutional care. *Social Problems,* **8,** 254–63.

SOMMER, R., WITNEY, G., and OSMOND, H. (1962). Teaching common associations to schizophrenics. *J. Abnorm. Soc. Psychol.* **65,** 58–61.

STANTON, A. H., and SCHWARTZ, M. S. (1954). *The mental hospital.* New York: Basic Books.

STOLLER, R. J., and GEERTSMA, R. H. (1963). The consistency of psychiatrists' clinical judgments. *J. Nerv. Ment. Dis.* **137,** 58–66.

STONE, R. C. (1958). The sociology of bureaucracy and professions. In J. S. ROUCEK (Ed.) *Contemporary sociology.* New York: Philosophical Library, 491–507.

STOTLAND, E., and KOBLER, A. L. (1965). *Life and death of a mental hospital.* Seattle, Wash.: Univer. of Washington Press.

STRASSMAN, H. D., THALER, M. B., and SCHEIN, E. H. (1956). A prisoner of war syndrome: apathy as a reaction to severe stress. *Amer. J. Psychiat.* **112,** 998–1003.

STRAUSS, A., SCHATZMAN, L., BUCHER, R., EHRLICH, D., and SABSHIN, M. (1964). *Psychiatric ideologies and institutions.* New York: the Free Press of Glencoe.

STRAUSS, A., SCHATZMAN, L., EHRLICH, D., BUCHER, R., and SABSHIN, M. (1963). The hospital and its negotiated order. In E. FREIDSON (Ed.) *The hospital in modern society.* New York: the Free Press of Glencoe, 147–69.

STUMPF, J. C. (1964). Two facets of psychiatric hospital effectiveness. In Symposium: An assessment of psychiatric hospital effectiveness. Amer. Psychol. Assoc. Convention, Los Angeles.

SZASZ, T. S. (1961). *The myth of mental illness.* New York: Hoeber Division of Harper & Row.

SZASZ, T. S. (1963). *Law, liberty, and psychiatry.* New York: Macmillan.

TALLACHI, S. (1960). Organization size, individual attitudes and behavior: an empirical study. *Admin. Sci. Quart.* **5,** 398–420.

TAYLOR, D. W., and FAUST, W. L. (1952). Twenty questions: efficiency of problem-solving as a function of group size. *J. Exp. Psychol.* **44,** 360–8.

TERRIEN, F. W., and MILLS, D. L. (1955). The effect of changing size upon the internal structure of organizations. *Amer. Sociol. Rev.* **20,** 11–13.

THOMAS, E. J. (1959). Role conceptions and organizational size. *Amer. Sociol. Rev.* **24,** 30–37.

THOMAS, E. J., and Fink, C. F. (1963). The effects of group size. *Psychol. Bull.* **60,** 371–84.

THOMPSON, V. A. (1963). *Modern organization.* New York: Knopf.

THORPE, L. P., and KATZ, B. (1948). *The psychology of abnormal behavior.* New York: Ronald Press.

TOCH, H. (1965). *The social psychology of social movements.* Indianapolis: Bobbs-Merrill.

TURNER, R. H. (1947). The navy disbursing officer as bureaucrat. *Amer. Sociol. Rev.* **12,** 342–8.

UDY, S. H., JR. (1959). "Bureaucracy" and "rationality" in Weber's organizational theory: an empirical study. *Amer. Sociol. Rev.* **24,** 791–5.

ULLMANN, L. P. (1961). Untestability of schizophrenics upon admission to psychiatric hospitals. *J. Clin. Psychol.* **17,** 199–202.

ULLMANN, L. P. (1965). A discussion of hospital social atmosphere profiles and their relevance to effectiveness. *J. Consult. Psychol.* **29,** 277–8.

ULLMANN, L. P., and BERKMAN, V. C. (1959a). Efficacy of placement of neuropsychiatric patients in family care. *Arch. Gen. Psychiat.* **1,** 273–4.

ULLMANN, L. P., and BERKMAN, V. C. (1959b). Judgments of outcome of home care placement from psychological material. *J. Clin. Psychol.* **15,** 28–31.

ULLMANN, L. P., and BERKMAN, V. C. (1959c). Types of outcome found in the family-care placement of mental patients. *Social Work,* **4,** 72–78.

ULLMANN, L. P., BERKMAN, V. C., and HAMISTER, R. C. (1958). Psychological reports related to behavior and benefit of placement in home care. *J. Clin. Psychol.* **14,** 254–9.

ULLMANN, L. P., FORSMAN, R. G., KENNY, J. W., MCINNIS, T. L., JR., UNIKEL, I. P., and ZEISSET, R. M. (1965). Selective reinforcement of schizophrenics' interview responses. *Behav. Res. Ther.* **2,** 205–12.

ULLMANN, L. P., and HUNRICHS, W. A. (1958). The role of anxiety in psychodiagnosis: replication and extension. *J. Clin. Psychol.* **14,** 276–9.

ULLMANN, L. P., and KRASNER, L. (Eds.) (1965). *Case studies in behavior modification.* New York: Holt, Rinehart, Winston.

ULLMANN, L. P., KRASNER, L., and COLLINS, B. J. (1961). Modification of behavior through verbal conditioning: effects in group therapy. *J. Abnorm. Soc. Psychol.* **62,** 128–32.

ULLMANN, L. P., KRASNER, L., and EDINGER, R. L. (1964). Verbal conditioning of common associations in long-term schizophrenic patients. *Behav. Res. Ther.* **2,** 15–18.

ULLMANN, L. P., WEISS, R. L., and KRASNER, L. (1963). The effect of verbal conditioning of emotional words on recognition of threatening stimuli. *J. Clin. Psychol.* **19,** 182–3.

U.S. DEPARTMENT OF HEALTH, EDUCATION, AND WELFARE (1963). Translation—the placebo problem. *Psychopharm. Serv. Center Bull.* **2** (No. 8, July), 1–65.

VON MERING, O., and KING, S. H. (1957). *Remotivating the mental patient.* New York: Russell Sage Foundation.

Vroom, V. H., and Maier, N. R. F. (1961). Industrial social psychology. In P. R. Farnsworth, O. McNemar, and Q. McNemar (Eds.) *Annual review of psychology* (Vol. 12). Stanford, Calif.: Annual Reviews, Inc., 413–46.

Wadsworth, W. V., Tonge, W. L., and Barber, L. E. (1957). The cost of treatment of affective disorders: a comparison between three mental hospitals. *Lancet*, **273** (Sept. 14), 534–5.

Walk, A. (1954). Some aspects of the "Moral Treatment" of the insane up to 1854. *J. Ment. Sci.* **100,** 807–37.

Walker, N. (1961). *Morale in the civil service.* Edinburgh: Edinburgh Univer. Press.

Wallace, A. F. C., and Rashkis, H. A. (1959). The relation of staff consensus to patient disturbance on mental hospital wards. *Amer. Sociol. Rev.* **24,** 829–35.

Wanklin, J. M., Fleming, D. F., Buck, C., and Hobbs, G. E. (1956). Discharge and readmissions among mental hospital patients. *Arch. Neurol. Psychiat.* **76,** 660–9.

Weiss, R. L., Krasner, L., and Ullmann, L. P. (1963). Responsivity of psychiatric patients to verbal conditioning: "success" and "failure" conditions and pattern of reinforced trials. *Psychol. Rep.* **12,** 423–6.

Werner, H. (1948). *Comparative psychology of mental development* (rev. ed.). Chicago: Follett.

Wessen, A. F. (1951). The social structure of a modern hospital. Unpublished doctoral dissertation, Yale Univer.

Wherry, R. J. (1948). What coordination is necessary? *Personnel Psychol.* **1,** 7–20.

Whyte, W. H., Jr. (1957). *The organization man.* Garden City, N.Y.: Doubleday.

Wilmer, H. A. (1958). *Social psychiatry in action.* Springfield, Ill.: Chas. C. Thomas.

Wilson, D. P., Knapp, S. C., Dondis, E., and Feder, Y. G. (1964). Course of mental illness in candidates for state hospitalization. *Calif. Ment. Hlth. Res. Dig.* **2** (No. 2, Spring), 40–42.

Wing, J. K., and Brown, G. W. (1961). Social treatment of chronic schizophrenia: a comparative study of three mental hospitals. *J. Ment. Sci.* **107,** 847–61.

Wittenborn, J., Holzberg, J., and Simon, B. (1953). Symptom correlates for descriptive diagnosis. *Genet. Psychol. Monogr.* **47,** 237–301.

Worthy, J. C. (1950). Organizational structure and employee morale. *Amer. Sociol. Rev.* **15,** 169–79.

Yates, A. J. (1958). Symptoms and symptom substitution. *Psychol. Rev.* **65,** 371–4.

Zander, A., Cohen, A. R., and Stotland, E. (1957), in collaboration with Hymovitch, B., and Riedl, O. *Role relations in the mental health professions.* Ann Arbor, Mich.: Institute for Social Research, University of Michigan.

Zigler, E., and Phillips, L. (1961). Psychiatric diagnosis and symptomatology. *J. Abnorm. Soc. Psychol.* **63,** 69–75.

Zilboorg, G., and Henry, G. W. (1941). *A history of medical psychology.* New York: Norton.

Zimet, C. N., and Brackbill, G. A. (1956). The role of anxiety in psychodiagnosis. *J. Clin. Psychol.* **12,** 173–7.

Zubin, J. (1953). Evaluation of therapeutic outcome in mental disorders. *J. Nerv. Ment. Dis.* **117,** 95–111.

# Index